D1466072

DEFENSE AGAINST ALZHEIMER'S DISEASE (DAAD)

A *RATIONAL* BLUEPRINT FOR PREVENTION

H. J. ROBERTS, M.D., F.A.C.P., F.C.C.P.

Active Staff, Good Samaritan Hospital and St. Mary's Hospital, West Palm Beach, Florida; Director, Palm Beach Institute for Medical Research, West Palm Beach; Diplomate, American Board of Internal Medicine (recertified); Medical Advisory Board, Alzheimer's Association of Palm Beach County; Member or Fellow - American College of Physicians, American College of Chest Physicians, The Endocrine Society, American Academy of Neurology, American Diabetes Association, American Heart Association, American Federation for Clinical Research, New York Academy of Sciences, American Association for the Advancement of Science, Sigma Xi (honor scientific research society), Alpha Omega Alpha (honor medical society); listed in *The Best Doctors In The U.S., Who's Who in America; Who's Who In The World, Who's Who In Frontier Science and Technology.*

Sunshine Sentinel Press, Inc.
West Palm Beach, Florida 33407

"To Inform and To Warn"

Publisher's Cataloging in Publication
(Prepared by Quality Books Inc.)

Roberts, H. J.
Defense against Alzheimer's disease (DAAD): a rational
blueprint for prevention/H. J. Roberts
p. cm.
Includes bibliographical references and index.
Preassigned LCCN: 93-086995.
ISBN 1-884243-00-2

1. Alzheimer's disease–Popular works. 2. Alzheimer's disease–
Prevention—Popular works. 1. Title.
RC523.R63 1994   616.8'31
                                  QB193-22661

The information in this book is not intended as a substitute for medical advice.
A physician should be consulted about questions or problems relating to any
of the matters considered.

Printed in the United States of America

Sunshine Sentinel Press, Inc.
P.O. Box 8697
West Palm Beach, FL 33407
FAX (407) 832-2400

CONTENTS

OTHER BOOKS BY THE WRITER

Difficult Diagnosis: A Guide to the Interpretation of Obscure Illness
    W. B. Saunders, Philadelphia, 1958

The Causes, Ecology and Prevention of Traffic Accidents
    Charles C Thomas, Springfield, 1971

Is Vasectomy Safe? Medical, Public Health and Legal Implications
    Sunshine Academic Press, West Palm Beach, 1979

Aspartame (NutraSweet®): Is It Safe?
    The Charles Press, Philadelphia, 1990

Sweet'ner Dearest: Bittersweet Vignettes About Aspartame (NutraSweet®)
    Sunshine Sentinel Press, West Palm Beach, 1992

Is Vasectomy Worth the Risk? A Physician's Case Against Vasectomania
    Sunshine Sentinel Press, West Palm Beach, 1993

A Guide to Personal Peace: The Control of Stress, Worry, Depression and Anxiety
    (Set of three cassettes). Sunshine Sentinel Press, West Palm Beach, 1993

Mega Vitamin E: Is It Safe?
    Sunshine Sentinel Press, West Palm Beach, 1994

West Palm Beach: Centennial Reflections
    Sunshine Sentinel Press, West Palm Beach, 1994

DEDICATION

This book is dedicated in gratitude to

Beatrice Trum Hunter

for her invaluable insights in many areas of
nutrition, health and general culture

ACKNOWLEDGEMENTS

Shirley Brightwell and Kathleen Brightwell	For excellent secretarial services.
Beatrice Trum Hunter and Esther Sokol	For valuable editing and suggestions.
Janice C. Cromar of Productions Unlimited, Inc.	For gracious assistance in the electronic prepress of the manuscript.
Susan Starr	For creating the front cover illustration.
Helen Musgrave, my office nurse for 35 years (!)	For assistance in managing many patients who developed Alzheimer's disease.
The librarian staffs at Good Samaritan Hospital and St. Mary's Hospital, West Palm Beach	For help in obtaining and checking references.
Muriel Brenner	For financial assistance.

I am indebted to the following persons and companies that granted permission to reproduce excerpts, figures, tables and cartoons:

American Diabetes Association (*Diabetes Care*)
Annals of Internal Medicine
The Boston Globe
Consumers' Research
Curtis Management Group (Figure by Dr. Frank H. Netter)
Earon S. Davis, Esq.
F. A. Davis Company (publisher of *Old Age Deterred* by Arnold Lorand)
Geriatric Medicine Today
HarperCollins Publishers
Ms. Beatrice Trum Hunter
Dr. Bradley T. Hyman
The Lancet
Dr. Lita Lee
Dr. Eugene H. Man
Modern Medicine
Neurology
New England Journal of Medicine
Dr. Nicholas Petkas
Roche Medical Image & Community
Mr. Jack Samuels
Dr. Adrienne Samuels
Southern Medical Journal
Dr. Robert Terry
The University of Chicago Press

To know how to grow old is the masterwork of wisdom,
and one of the most difficult chapters
in the great art of living.

Henri Amiel
(*Journal Intime* 1874)

But the interesting thing – or better, the tragedy – is that the
most dangerous things we do, and our most dangerous
items, provoke no fear at all. We decide caveat emptor
*when, but only when, it is convenient to do so.**

Dr. John B. Thomison (1983)

The rational development of therapy for a disease depends
critically on knowledge about its pathogenesis. In the
absence of such insight, physicians are vulnerable to
the prevailing winds of opinion and practice, each
*liable to shift from one moment to another***

Dr. William B. Rizzo (1993)

Today there is neither a cure nor a treatment that can stop the
progression or reverse the course of the intellectual decline.
A diagnosis of Alzheimer's disease today carries with it
a sentence of eventual mental emptiness.

U.S. Department of Health and Human Services
Task Force on Alzheimer's Disease (1984)

DISCLAIMERS

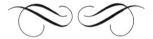

PREFACE AND OVERVIEW

A man's real possession is his memory.

Alexander Smith

I have but one lamp by which my feet are guided: and that is the lamp of experience. I know of no way of judging the future but by the past.

Patrick Henry
(Speech to the Virginia Convention, 1775)

I will call attention to one fact, apparent to anyone familiar with the history of medical discoveries: that the relative value of such discoveries bears not the slightest relation to the rapidity of acceptance by the medical profession.

Dr. William B. Coley

All Americans must be shaken, and saddened, by news that former President Ronald Reagan is battling with Alzheimer's Disease... Unfortunately, this disease still has no effective treatment, and no means of prevention. But to borrow one of President Reagan's favorite metaphors, the dawn of discovery in neuroscience is beginning to lift the darkness of this dread disease.

David Mahoney
Chairman, The Dana Alliance for Brain Initiatives
(November 8, 1994)

DEFENSE AGAINST ALZHEIMER'S DISEASE (DAAD) represents a unique project by one physician... perhaps the first attempted on such a panoramic scale. It offers the general reader insights aimed at preventing, delaying or minimizing the threat of Alzheimer's disease (AD). This work is the result of an "agonizing reappraisal" to unravel a disorder which some have designated as "the cruelest disease" in this "Age of Age," and to preserve so-called "working" or "vital" memory.

AD now constitutes a medical, social and economic scourge. This relentless and dehumanizing affliction destroys memory and personality, and ultimately causes or accelerates death. Numerous anecdotes attest to the dramatic awareness of dementia by a spouse—for example, the inability of a brilliant individual, previously described as a "walking dictionary," to remember simple words.

The fact that Alzheimer's disease is a 20th Century phenomenon provides an additional sobering perspective. Specifically, Dr. Alois Alzheimer reported the single case of a 51-year-old German woman in 1907. The significance of this time and place relates directly to a question being universally asked by relatives and caregivers of AD patients: "Why has our society been victimized by this disease?"

I shall emphasize certain clinical features and changes in body physiology that could appear to signal "early," "evolving" or "transitional" AD. Accordingly, "SUSPECT ALZHEIMER'S!" in the appropriate setting is the message, especially for persons who have certain "risk factors."

The AD-prone state evolves from the effects of multiple risk factors. It is NOT solely "genetic." Awareness of these factors becomes paramount if preventive measures (Section IV) are to be instituted BEFORE an irreversible amount of brain damage occurs. Stated differently, a multifaceted approach is required to protect the brain and to rescue its damaged functional activities during the long phase that generally *precedes* dementia... probably 20-30 years in the majority of cases!

This book *specifically* focuses on preventing AD. It therefore does not deal with the treatment of patients having the advanced disease. Numerous books on that aspect are available for health professionals, relatives and caregivers. However, some of the measures cited in Section IV might benefit persons with "early" AD before gross deterioration has occurred. These include insuring adequate nutrition and oxygen to the brain, and avoiding further exposure to common neurotoxins known to be present in food, water and the environment.

THE URGENT NEED FOR PUBLICATION

A sense of urgency led me to condense many observations and years of research for the general reader, and place a higher priority for publishing this book than my larger scientific text on AD. I continue to be impressed by the near-universal interest of intelligent persons in this subject, and their thirst for sensible measures that might prevent AD. A quip is pertinent in this context: "Some diseases are too important to be left only in the hands of doctors and researchers."

The following considerations also influenced my decision to prioritize this book:

- AD is escalating at an alarming rate not only in the aged, but also among maturing "baby boomers." More than four million persons in the United States already have this disease. As a basis for comparison, AD currently afflicts 18 times more individuals in Florida than AIDS—specifically, 288,623 cases in October 1991, compared to 15,726 cases of AIDS (*The Miami Herald* October 20, 1991, p. C-1).

- An estimated 250,000 new cases of symptomatic AD are occurring annually.

- One out of three families in the United States has experienced the destabilizing impact caused by AD in a member.

- As many as two-thirds of family caregivers suffer severe depression as a result of becoming "secondary hostages" to this form of bondage. They must shoulder the economic burden if eligibility for Medicaid has not been met.

- The public is continually exposed to numerous neurotoxins capable of destroying brain cells. Industry introduces some 1,000 new chemicals every year, generally without information (known or suspected) about their potential long-term hazards for humans. Similarly, many food additives and supplements legally classified "Generally Recognized As Safe" (GRAS) by the Food and Drug Administration (FDA) continue in use without definitive clarification of published suspicions about their safety — that is, the evaluation of extensive data on humans by corporate-neutral investigators.

- Ideas about preventing, delaying or minimizing the misery of AD will be rejected by most physicians if they cannot be furnished <u>absolute</u> proof of its cause(s)... even in the face of considerable incriminating or suggestive evidence.

- It is unlikely that any pharmacologic "magic bullet" can "cure" AD in the wake of sufficient nerve cell death to have caused dementia.

- Primary emphasis upon prevention for the population at risk must be based on reasonable attempts to avoid or correct neurotoxic influences <u>before</u> advanced neurological deterioration has occurred.

Any skeptic who doubts the urgency of this mandate should visit a nursing home where the majority of patients are being "warehoused" because they have AD. The dementia and related disabilities in their hoped-for "golden years" often contrast sharply with the joy and vigor that characterized their productive business, professional and social lives. This is particularly poignant in the case of individuals verging on genius, as occurred with Aaron Copeland and Maurice Ravel.

Paradoxically, many aging Americans blessed with increased longevity now fear the loss of control over their lives and "imprisonment" in a nursing home far more than sudden death. This theme repeatedly surfaces in the form of suicide or attempted suicide, and reports of homicide by a loving spouse-caregiver after demoralization by the chronic ordeal.

OVERVIEW OF THE BOOK

This book provides basic medical and scientific considerations that are essential both for understanding AD and the proposed blueprint of prophylaxis. "Medicalese" is minimized, when possible. But I also have heeded William Maxwell's advice to authors: "You must be aware that your reader is at least as bright as you are."

<u>Section I</u> summarizes the important clinical, epidemiologic and pathologic

(disease) aspects of AD. Any proposed cause(s) of AD should explain or clarify these phenomena.

Section II presents my current beliefs about the causation of AD, coupled with the essential supporting evidence. They encompass *common* medical, nutritional, environmental and technologic factors known to damage brain cells and to interfere with nerve function. By the time AD becomes manifest as a dementing disorder after decades of "evolving" AD, large numbers of vital brain cells have been destroyed.

Others are arriving at a similar conclusion about the multifactorial causation of AD. Blass (1993) aptly suggested the term "convergence syndrome" — or "the syndrome of the bits" — wherein various genetic and environmental abnormalities could effect the brain damage characteristic of this disease.

Section III lists major risk factors and neurotoxic influences, and the medical settings in which they may be found. They are the distillation of many clinical observations and extensive researches done in related fields by myself and others.

Section IV offers a prudent and reasonable approach to avoiding or minimizing such neurotoxicity. It is analogous to the current emphasis on preventing heart attacks by defining and countering "coronary risk factors." Given individual differences and circumstances, considerable variations are inevitable. Measures for coping with contributory stress appear in Chapter 19. They reflect the statement by Seneca: "Man does not die; he kills himself."

The Bibliography contains pertinent references from which others can be located.

EVOLUTION OF MY INTEREST IN ALZHEIMER'S DISEASE

My interest in AD—and those disorders that often precede or accompany it—evolved over more than three decades. I was particularly impressed by the development of severe confusion, memory loss, and inability to communicate in some patients whom I had doctored previously for other health problems.

Serendipity or fortunate coincidence also played a role. Some of my researches involving other medical disorders (e.g., multiple sclerosis, hypoglycemia, diabetes mellitus) unexpectedly came to figure prominently in crystallizing the AD-prone state. The confusion and memory loss associated with reactions to products containing aspartame (NutraSweet®) provided intriguing insights.

These circumstances served to catalyze new concepts about the causation of AD. Further observation and investigation have validated their pertinence.

In effect, this book describes such a "paradigm shift." (This evocative term was used by Thomas Kuhn [1970] to describe the wrenching change from one set of fundamental scientific beliefs to another.) Its goal is to age with intact brain function without invoking the joke that the only sure way of doing so is to die while young.

ABOUT THE AUTHOR

I graduated with honors from Tufts University College of Medicine, and have practiced as a Board-certified internist and medical consultant for more than 40 years.

For three decades, I have served as Director of the Palm Beach Institute for Medical Research. In this nonsalaried, corporate-neutral capacity, I had the opportunity of exploring a broad range of medical, nutritional, neurologic and environmental challenges.

I am a member of prestigious medical organizations and scientific societies—e.g., The Endocrine Society and the American Academy of Neurology.

My writings include seven books and more than 200 published articles and letters. Many are listed in the Bibliography. They encompass diagnosis, original forms of testing, and novel therapeutic approaches to challenging disorders.

ANTICIPATED CRITICISM FROM PHYSICIANS

It is fair to warn readers that many physicians are likely to criticize my views and recommendations. Some will flatly reject the notion that diet, habits, life style, neurotoxins and stress play contributory roles... largely because they have not been previously exposed to these ideas in the context of AD. This observation in 1888 by Jean-Martin Charcot, a famous neurologist, about the acceptance of new discoveries is germane:

> "Such was the case for so many other ideas which are today universally accepted because they are based on demonstrable evidence, but which met for so long only skepticism and often sarcasm—it is only a matter of time."

The major thrust of DAAD focuses upon two words in the title—"rational" and "prevention." Most neurologists and other physicians reflexively will challenge this assertion on several grounds. First, prevention presumably cannot be rational if a specific cause has not been unequivocally demonstrated. Second, to my knowledge no responsible physician heretofore has advanced any panoramic program aimed at preventing AD based on clinical and scientific evidence. Third, distinguished neurologists have deemphasized diagnosing the "early" diagnosis of AD because there is no effective treatment (Mark 1992). I disagree, especially when multiple risk factors can be identified.

I acknowledge the limitations of a single physician in such an undertaking, and the considerable study that will be required to prove some of the basic issues I raise. However, I bring to the subject considerable experience in dealing with these medical and societal realities. Oliver Wendell Holmes aptly remarked in a 1867 lecture to the medical class of Harvard University: "The bedside is always the true center of medical teaching."

Such anticipated criticism from "the establishment" warrants the following additional comments:

- Not every approach to AD has been sought or tried by physicians and scientists.

- A doctor or health professional who proposes prophylactic advice without providing definitive statistical data gathered at a major medical center can expect negative reactions. Unfortunately, this kind of ingrained thinking tends to inhibit progress. Samuel Johnson was familiar with such an attitude when he observed: "Nothing will ever be attempted if all possible objections must first be overcome."

- Excessive concentration on details of the advanced disease has tended to deemphasize the study of early causative factors, especially in the face of a "syndrome shift." This phenomenon is illustrated by a person with narcolepsy (severe sleepiness) who becomes involved in a traffic accident. Such an individual is likely to be treated only for the secondary injuries... not the primary cause of the mishap (falling asleep at the wheel).

ANTICIPATED CRITICISM FROM INDUSTRY

Criticism from representatives of industries having vested interests in potentially neurotoxic products is inevitable.

My views derive from close focus on common foods, food additives, drugs, chemicals and other technologic "advances" that had not been evaluated adequately in animals and humans before and after their marketing. Unfortunately, such risk is pervasive. Without more enlightened supervision by several key regulatory agencies, the "masks of deception" in promoting comparable products will continue.

Corporations understandably go to great lengths to protect their interests. This is all the more likely for products implicated in the causation of AD—directly or indirectly.Industry also must rebut the charge of "science for sale" if documentation of the alleged safety of certain products, both old and new, is demanded. They include additives (monosodium glutamate; aspartame), drugs (aluminum-containing antacids), chemicals (fluoride in toothpaste and water fluoridation; mercury-containing dental amalgam), and some forms of food processing (ultrapasteurization).

A fundamental issue is encompassed in this question: "When does the uninhibited pursuit of perceived technologic advances become overkill for our society relative to their neurologic, carcinogenic and other medical complications?" The title of an editorial in the *Journal of the American Medical Association* by Dr. William R. Hendee (1991) conveyed this theme: "There's No Free Lunch: The Benefits And Risks Of Technologies."

A CHALLENGE FOR THE READER

Seemingly healthy individuals who have had a family member or close friend afflicted with AD must avoid intimidation by the foregoing controversies. There is real hope for preventing or minimizing AD by concerned persons who have defined risk factors IF you and they are willing to do three things.

First, weigh the evidence yourself. No one has all the answers to this enigma... including me. But you can—and should—analyze legitimate data when your brain is at risk. At the very least, this effort will make you a more informed individual.

Second, extract those meaningful kernels of knowledge and advice that make sense, especially in conjunction with other insights concerning your body and health. They include details about members of the family, previous health experiences, dietary habits, a host of environmental factors that invite exposure to known neurotoxins, and even your personality.

Third, be willing to commit yourself *for years* to some form of ongoing DAAD program of constructive hygienic measures derived from suggestions in this book and your own study. In effect, you must become a true believer in such an effort at self-preservation. It is analogous to abstinence and other behavioral modifications by persons seeking to avoid HIV infection. Realize, too, that some skeptic is likely to ridicule any regimen by asserting that you probably will not develop AD. But stand firm.Does maintaining an accident-free record disturb you because you took the

14

proper precautions to drive safely?

For further orientation, I suggest that the unbiased general reader ask more questions.

- Ask the spouses and caregivers of AD patients if they would have pursued reasonable and harmless hygienic measures aimed at prevention had they known about them.

- Ask some prominent neurologist about the documented value of dozens of purported "magic bullets" for AD — including experimental drugs released by the FDA for reasons of compassion or political expediency. You will find that none have had a predictable "Lazarus effect," as depicted in the movie *Awakenings*. Alleged "breakthroughs" (all having enormously profitable commercial overtones) were based largely on slightly better recognition of familiar faces or improved sleep through the night.

Commitment to DAAD by thoughtful individuals can influence relatives and friends… and ultimately the community. It also may enhance the realization among doctors, scientists and business leaders that widespread exposures to neurotoxins in food, water and air DO threaten our *entire* society. This threat is as great as the drastic loss of ozone over the Antarctic, where there are no refrigerators or air conditioners releasing chlorofluorocarbons (CFSs) and fluorinated gases.

PERSONAL RESPONSIBILITY

Concerned adults ought to initiate efforts aimed at preventing Alzheimer's disease NOW. Admittedly, our knowledge of many issues about AD remains limited. But are you willing to wait while "experts" debate endlessly, and as risk factors keep increasing exponentially?

A German proverb embodies my message: "Every man is the locksmith of his own happiness." You are entitled to think, study, and act in your own best interest when it comes to proper care of the remarkable organ above your neck that has made you "human." Furthermore, taking this responsibility can benefit your children and other family members.

The desperate wish of most persons to "stay in control" was mentioned earlier. The vast majority of my patients are resigned to the fact they must depart sometime. But they also express the unequivocal wish to remain in control of their lives, and to make decisions up till the very end. That is probably why you are reading this book.

A physician who has reported the potential ramifications of first-hand observations and researches may wonder about such efforts until receiving unsolicited correspondence… even a single letter. This theme was contained in a feature published by *The Wall Street Journal* (February 28, 1994, p. B-1) titled, "Dear Author: Your Book Has Changed My Life."

The extreme emphasis on overspecialization has relevance to my previous comment that protection against major disease is too important to be entrusted solely to medical and public health professionals. A narrow professional focus tends to distort overall perspective concerning environmental factors, the human condition, and a host of related societal, technologic, economic and political issues.

15

DISCLAIMERS AND CAVEATS

Conscience and prudence dictate the following disclaimers and caveats:

- My suggestions are generic, and not intended as substitutes for medical advice. At the very least, they certainly qualify as "proper hygienic principles."

- Readers should seek a physician's opinion concerning any details that differ from medical recommendations. These may relate to the use of tranquilizers, aluminum-containing antacids, megadoses of vitamin E, fluoridated toothpaste, and even the choice of anesthetic agents. *The physician, however, must be knowledgeable about your reason for such concern, or make it his or her business to explore the matter.*

- I can give no guarantee that adherence to the general recommendations listed will prevent or retard the development of AD in a specific individual.

- There is no intent of malice or disrespect toward any manufacturer, producer, physician, researcher or organization whose products, studies or recommendations are discussed.

SECTION I

A REVIEW OF ALZHEIMER'S DISEASE

The truth is seldom pure and never simple.

Oscar Wilde

*Infirmity doth still neglect all office whereto our health is bound;
we are not ourselves when nature, being oppress'd,
commands the mind to suffer with the body.*

Shakespeare
(*King Lear* Act II, Scene IV)

For readers of this book who are not health care professionals, this section reviews the clinical features (Chapter 1), the pertinent statistics (Chapter 2), and changes found within the brain (Chapters 4 and 5) of Alzheimer's disease (AD) patients. It will help in understanding the components of a *rational* long-term program, detailed in Section IV, aimed at preventing or delaying its ravages.

The issue of heredity troubles many relatives of AD victims. It is considered in Chapter 3. Presently, I believe that any inherited component more likely either involves one or several generalized metabolic disorders to which the brain is uniquely vulnerable, or renders it more susceptible to diverse environmental insults.

The panoramic hypothesis concerning causation (Section II) and the various risk factors described in Section III provide further insights.

Historical Perspectives

Some historical background is germane. *Alzheimer's disease represents a disorder first encountered as a specific clinical <u>and</u> pathologic entity during the 20th Century.* There will be repeated reference to this fact as well as the basic question, "What changes introduced since about 1900 have been conducive to such degeneration of the brain?"

The single case reported by Alois Alzheimer appeared in a German medical periodical during 1907. It was titled, "Über Eine Eigenartige Erkrankung der Hirnride" ("About a Peculiar Disease of Cerebral Cortex"). At the age of 51, this woman became unreasonably suspicious of her husband. Dramatic impairment of memory ensued until her death four and one-half years later.

Two aspects of the report are noteworthy. First, the editors of this journal—astute physicians and scientists acknowledged as authorities in their fields—wrote the following preface: "The picture he presents is of a case so deviant even on clinical grounds alone that it does not fit into any of the known disease categories, and *the anatomical findings diverge from all currently known disease processes*" (translated from the German by L. Jarvik and H. Greenson for the Alzheimer's Association).

Admittedly, isolated descriptions of an AD-like dementing illness were noted by previous writers and physicians, but without the pathologic details provided by Alzheimer. A striking example can be found in *Gulliver's Travels* by the satirist Jonathan Swift, published in 1726 "to vex the world."

Second, the patient resided in Frankfurt/Main, where she had been institutionalized. Because Germany was at the forefront of chemical innovation, both industrial and pharmacologic, its population doubtless became exposed to novel environmental neurotoxins. These have increased exponentially as contaminants in water, air, food and drugs over subsequent decades… generally with little awareness or concern by the medical profession or regulatory agencies. Our society now is forced to confront one of the costs for such corporate-driven commercialism and uninhibited consumerism: an epidemic of Alzheimer's disease.

> A remarkable coincidence occurred in discussing the cover design with Susan Starr, a graphic artist. I happened to mention Alzheimer's case and the city wherein she resided. Susan exclaimed, "My grandmother had Alzheimer's disease—and she was born and lived in Frankfurt/Main!"

A 20th Century Milestone

The circa 1900 era warrants further comment here, and will be repeatedly mentioned in subsequent chapters.

Enormous changes were being thrust upon an increasingly urban society at the turn of the 20th Century. They resulted from the combination of scientific-technologic discovery and intensive industrial energy, coupled with economic entrepreneurship. Astute observers already began expressing concern over this state of affairs. Henry Adams brilliantly expounded on this theme in his "Law of Acceleration (1904)" (*The Education of Henry Adams,* 1918).

Adams marveled that a six-year-old boy "born into a new world" had seen the fruition of the railway, the ocean steamer, the electric telegraph, the Daguerreotype, and the increase of coal output in the United States to over 300 million tons. But he reflected that this compulsive course was causing Nature to revolt violently "every day… while plainly laughing at man." There is no more convincing evidence for such "laughter" than the dementia attributable to technological "progress" described in this book.

1

SYMPTOMS AND SIGNS

*Observation is more than seeing; it is knowing what you see
and comprehending its significance. The process is far
more mental than photographic. True observation
implies studying the object and drawing
conclusions from what is seen.*

Charles Gow

*All the business of war, and indeed all the business of life,
is to endeavour to find out what you don't know by
what you do; that's what I call "guessing what
is on the other side of the hill."*

Arthur Wellesley, Duke of Wellington

Advanced Alzheimer's disease (AD) is characterized by severe confusion, memory loss, inability to concentrate or reason, slowed speech and thought, difficulty in maintaining a conversation, impaired handwriting, a gross change in personality, and progressive deterioration. It is not part of the "normal aging process."

Although also referred to as senile dementia of the Alzheimer's type (SDAT), individuals in their 50s or younger can be victimized. This relentless affliction has terminated many productive business, professional and social careers. It becomes particularly poignant in the case of highly gifted persons (see Preface).

The overt dementia of AD is probably preceded in most instances by longstanding general and neuropsychiatric features. Indeed, most neuropathologists now believe that extensive changes exist for decades within the brains of AD patients (Chapter 4). Accordingly, physicians and others must adopt a "THINK ALZHEIMER'S!" mindset

20

when confronted with unexplained clinical features noted here and in Section III. Progression of the brain damage might be minimized and delayed by detecting such clinical clues and risk factors relatively early, and then instituting measures to counter both causative and contributory factors. That is the purpose of this book.

CLINICAL FEATURES OF ALZHEIMER'S DISEASE

"Dementia" is a behavioral diagnosis. It describes severely impaired intellectual function that interferes with the pursuit of one's occupation and social activities. Dementia also implies the absence of altered consciousness. Owing to the numerous and contradictory implications of "dementia," Hachinski (1992) suggested the term "dysmentia."

Other evidences of impaired brain function may accompany or precede dementia in AD patients. They can be obvious or highly subtle. Some are reviewed below and in Section III.

- The "anxiety" of patients with evolving AD may resemble the anxiety in persons experiencing severe stress and exhaustion.

- The vague complaint, "I just don't feel like myself," is frequently voiced by these patients. It could signify loss of enthusiasm, diminished creativity, disinterest in favorite pastimes, or the inability to express affection.

Severe dementia largely relates to the extent and duration of changes within the brain (Chapters 4 and 5). However, *extensive degeneration already exists at the "early" symptomatic stage of AD.*

Dementia

The dementing features frequently encountered in AD victims include confusion, an inability to recall, difficulty in speech, altered judgment and impaired abstract thinking. A highly sensitive indicator of "early" AD is markedly delayed recall of words, time, place and persons—that is, after allowing a lapse of many minutes.

Many subtleties are involved. Persons with evolving AD whose basic personality remains intact not infrequently compensate for significant memory loss through denial and other tactics. Spouses, friends and even doctors are often amazed at the extent of dementia when such individuals become acutely ill, or "get lost" while driving a car or walking in their neighborhood. For example, *42 percent of 208 demented patients in a large community survey were not recognized as being demented by their personal physicians* (O'Connor 1988)!

Denial is common when the individual continues to hold a job and interact socially. At this stage, he or she can readily rationalize the forgetting of seldom-used names and phone numbers. The mechanisms used for deflecting suspicion include confabulation (making up stories), maintaining social graces ("tea party dementia"), and laughing off or dodging demanding questions. A spouse who attempts to compensate for such impairment might be compounding the problem.

Advanced AD probably exists if the person repeatedly fails to remember the place, the previous sentence of a conversation, his or her birthday and age, the names of family members, the current president, or how to make change... especially when given sufficient time as noted above. Failure to recognize a spouse is even more significant.

A number of "scientific" tests are used to confirm mental deterioration. They focus on deficits in the realms discussed above, the ability to calculate, and the comprehension of simple jokes, sayings and cartoons.

The so-called <u>Mini-Mental State Examination</u> is commonly used for mental and functional assessment, especially in differentiating dementia from depression, and to monitor patients over time. The test requires about 10 minutes, and can be administered in a primary-care setting. The functional testing includes orientation, registration of simple information, attention, calculation, recall, language and copying. The details can be found in most neurology texts and books on AD.

Language and Related Disturbances

Brain dysfunction in evolving AD often involves language in its diverse ramifications. Some examples:

- inability to find the correct word
- perseveration in speech by using more "filler" words
- circumlocution (talking around the subject)
- inability to express one's thoughts in writing
- inability to understand written language (even though the ability to read words may be retained)
- inability to transmit a message from the brain to the fingers or feet for carrying out a command (apraxia), as evidenced by difficulty in performing customary activities—e.g., unlocking a door with a key; dramatic deterioration of handwriting or gait; inability to dial a telephone number

Other Behavioral Clues

"THINK ALZHEIMER'S!" should be triggered by the following clues suggesting an "organic personality disorder." Severe intellectual impairment, however, may <u>not</u> be evident at the time.

- deterioration of personal hygiene (e.g., reluctance to bathe or shower)
- inappropriate dress in public
- total disarray in the home of an individual who lives alone
- sloppiness with one's personal appearance or work
- inability to complete work in the usual time
- showing up for appointments at the wrong time
- losing or misplacing things
- repeated traffic accidents caused by inability to resolve unexpected encounters or problems in a timely manner (Friedland 1988)
- the loss of "social graces"
- withdrawal or disinterest as manifest by apathy, loss of spontaneity, or inability to start anything new
- irritability
- stubbornness
- tactlessness
- repeated questioning or complaining
- inappropriate silliness
- suspiciousness (e.g., accusing a spouse or children of theft or infidelity)

- uncharacteristic cursing
- obsessive attention to trivial things (e.g., locks; dust; garbage)
- buying items that already were purchased
- difficulty in shopping and handling money
- a short attention span for visiting or for watching television
- a change in sexual appetite or performance
- inability to follow instructions, written or oral

Comments on "Normal Aging"

The significance of some minor decrease in mental function that accompanies "normal aging" should not be exaggerated. One aspect involves "executive function"—a term used by neuroscientists for describing the ability of an individual to perform several tasks at the same time, or to rapidly switch back and forth between tasks. The individual often can overcome such a slight decline through better organization of work in order to focus on one task at a time.

Similarly, the inability to locate misplaced glasses or keys, or one's car on a parking lot, ought not cause panic through their misinterpretation as an "early warning signal" of AD. The same applies to brief lapses in recalling a word or a name. In some instances, the inference of failing memory by a successful person only may be relative. For example, an impatient spouse, child or business associate might be reflexively giving the answer without allowing the individual sufficient time for recollection.

Individuals can perform various do-it-yourself tests in deciding whether the perceived loss of memory represents a serious cognitive problem. Some examples:

- Recollect the frequency of forgetting where one's car was parked in a parking lot.
- Attempt to repeat a list of 8 or 10 common words that are read by someone.
- Identify common objects in pictures shown by someone.
- Attempt to mime some familiar activity, such as initiating driving or lighting a cigarette, in order to determine whether the sequence of steps is both proper and appropriate.

A few errors should not be considered grossly abnormal. On the other hand, a significant number of errors warrants professional consultation.

The "failure to thrive" of elderly persons, also referred to as "the dwindles," is not an aspect of normal aging. It should initiate a search for causes other than AD that are treatable or preventable (see below). They include malnutrition, various medical diseases, the use of alcohol and drugs, severe sensory deficits, depression, and a host of socioeconomic problems that culminate in despair ("the giving-up complex").

DIAGNOSIS

The diagnosis of AD or probable Alzheimer's disease (PAD) is generally correct when other causes of dementia have been excluded both on clinical grounds and by appropriate studies. This was the case in 88 percent of 294 confirmed cases in one study (Mendez 1991b). The incorrect diagnoses chiefly included multi-infarct disease (multiple small strokes), Binswanger's disease, Parkinson's disease, primary depression (pseudodementia), and alcoholic dementia.

> Binswanger's disease is also referred to as "border zone infarction" because small strokes tend to occur at the borders between areas supplied by two major arteries to the brain (the anterior cerebral artery and the middle cerebral artery). It is likely to complicate a severe or repeated drop in blood pressure from the overaggressive treatment of hypertension.

Specific attention must be directed to potentially treatable conditions that can present as dementia. They include an underactive thyroid (hypothyroidism), the side effects of drugs (both prescription and over-the-counter), vitamin B-12 deficiency, increased fluid within the brain's cavities or ventricles (normal-pressure hydrocephalus), and certain infections (e.g., syphilis).

- The components of over-the-counter cold remedies can result in severe confusion—e.g., dextromethorphan in popular cough preparations (e.g., Robitussin DM®).

- Chronic inflammatory meningoencephalitis, another dementing illness, must be considered in the differential diagnosis because of the remarkable response of dementia to oral corticosteroid therapy (Caselli 1993). The presence of Sjögren's syndrome—characterized by dry mouth, dry eyes (due to decreased tears), increased deep tendon reflexes, an unsteady gait, Babinski signs (elevation of the great toe on stroking the bottom of the foot), and the presence of Sjögren's antibodies—provides an important clue to this potentially treatable disorder.

Diligent diagnostic effects may be required. For instance, tests of the cerebrospinal fluid for syphilis may be positive when serologic blood tests are negative.

There are other diagnostic caveats. As a case in point, the diagnosis of AD should not be based solely on the finding of "brain atrophy" by computed tomography (CT) or magnetic resonance imaging (MRI) studies.

Pseudodementia due to Depression

This diagnosis ALWAYS must be considered in older persons because it may respond dramatically to conventional therapy. However, true dementia might develop later in a depressed patient with pseudodementia (Kral 1989; Chapter 15). This is suggested by the continuing decline in intellectual function after seemingly successful treatment of depression.

A vicious cycle of memory loss can occur when minor degrees of forgetfulness result in superimposed depression… with the associated difficulty in concentration and decreased attention span. Under these circumstances, sensitive persons may panic in the belief they are replicating a parent's loss of mental faculties once they reach one of the "big zeros"—usually 50 or 60 years.

The possibility of underlying depression must be explored even in individuals who have been institutionalized for a presumed diagnosis of dementia, particularly when based largely on inability to concentrate. The problem can be compounded in older persons through the aggressive administration of tranquilizers and sedatives (Chapter 11). Diligent probing may uncover precipitating factors relating to finances, the lack of attention by children, and drastic changes in housing. Experienced physicians have observed dramatic improvement in memory when such problems were discussed and resolved.

Criteria for the Diagnosis of "Probable Alzheimer's Disease" (PAD)

Recurrent or persistent impairment of memory resulting in drastic consequences warrants medical consultation for the proper diagnosis of PAD. To repeat some examples:

- Confusion concerning the place or the time
- Inability to name familiar objects
- Gross problems when driving—e.g., failure to observe a one-way sign; becoming lost in one's neighborhood
- Failure to recall important appointments
- Failure to remember having told the same story to the same person(s)
- Inability to utilize one's previous ability in math, simple accounting, music or other skills

Table 1-1 lists the criteria that are usually acceptable for making a diagnosis of "probable Alzheimer's disease." At least two features of cognitive dysfunction should be present.

TABLE 1-1

CRITERIA FOR THE CLINICAL DIAGNOSIS OF PROBABLE ALZHEIMER'S DISEASE

Progressive deterioration in two or more areas of cognitive function (language, motor skills, perception) without a disturbance of consciousness or contributory drugs
Dementia may be established on clinical examination by the Mini-Mental State Examination or similar testing, and neuro-psychologic studies
Impaired activities of daily living
Altered patterns of behavior
Onset after age 40
Most often in the 60s
A family history of a dementing disorder
Evidence of cerebral and hippocampal atrophy (loss of nerve cells) by CT or MRI imaging studies (Chapter 4)
Absence of an acute onset
Absence of focal neurologic findings
E.g., muscle weakness; sensory loss; visual field deficits; incoordination early in the course of the illness
Absence of systemic disorders or other brain diseases that could account for progressive deterioration of memory and cognition (see above)
Normal cerebrospinal fluid studies (by standard techniques)
Normal electroencephalographic (brain wave) pattern or non-specific changes (such as increased slow-wave activity)
Coexistence of relevant conditions (Chapters 15 and 16)
E.g., Parkinson's disease

The detection of memory dysfunction in "very early" AD could be crucial relative to minimizing or delaying severe dementia by addressing risk factors that are found. At this early stage, the best discriminator appears to be some measure(s) of learning that involve acquisition and recall with semantic cuing—comparable to tests of function for other organs using exercise or stress (Petersen 1994).

2

EPIDEMIOLOGY AND STATISTICS

*Dementia as a public health problem looms
as the epidemic of the 21st century.*

Dr. L. Bachman et al (1992)

*Old age can sometimes seem like a punishment at the end of
even an exemplary life. Here in the USA, 40% of men and
women aged 75 and over will sink into dementia, mostly
from Alzheimer's disease, before they die.*

J. B. Sibbison (1991)

Alzheimer's disease (AD) constitutes an unequivocal epidemic. Yet, neither clinicians nor pathologists recognized this disease before 1907 (Introduction to Section I).

AD or probable AD accounts for more than half of the patients with severe dementia in our society. Furthermore, it now represents the fourth leading cause of death among adults, more than 100,000 persons succumbing to it annually.

Number of Cases

The following data reinforce the magnitude of this affliction in the United States.

- AD currently affects more than four million persons.

- An estimated 250,000 new cases are being diagnosed annually.

- As of April 1991, the Alzheimer's Association of Palm Beach County had a patient load of 12,000 persons with a physician-diagnosis of probable AD (Chapter 1).

- The number of individuals 65 and older will double by the year 2030, thereby constituting 20 percent of the population (Wecker 1991).

27

- An estimated 14 million "Baby Boomer" Americans will be afflicted with AD by the year 2040.

AD is plaguing other "developed" counties, too. A EURODEM Concerted Action Study reported the progressively higher incidence of this disease across Europe (Rocca 1991). The overall prevalence (per 100 population) for the age groups 30-59, 60-69, 70-79, and 80-89 was 0.02, 0.3, 3.1, and 10.8, respectively.

A 25-year time trend study in Rochester (Minnesota) (Kokmen 1993b), encompassing 1960-1984, indicated a definite change in the incidence of dementing illness. The proportion of cases attributed to dementia of unknown cause decreased, while the proportion of cases due to AD increased, especially in the older age groups—amounting to 2,600/100,000 person years for the oldest age group.

The Social and Economic Toll

The social and economic havoc caused by AD has been catastrophic in virtually every community. The progressive dependency of its victims imposes an enormous responsibility and drain upon spouses, children, relatives, friends, health care professionals, and social services organizations. For example:

- A conservative estimate of the present annual cost of AD in the United States is $88 billion.
- One out of three families has had a member ravaged by this disease.
- Two-thirds of caregivers are believed to suffer severe depression as a result of the physical, emotional and economic strain, particularly when they receive minimal or no personal assistance and monetary help. Most are spouses and daughters (Mohide 1993).
- AD patients fill more than 50 percent of the beds in most nursing homes—at an annual cost of more than $25 billion.
- The current annual cost of formal and informal care per AD patient is as high as $47,000 (Max 1993).
- The Florida Department of Elder Affairs has been able to meet the needs of only *one percent* (!) of the State's 288,000 AD patients (Lipscomb 1991).

Traffic Accidents

AD contributes significantly to traffic accidents through impaired driving due to reduced attention span, altered judgment, and a slow reaction time (O'Neill 1992). The accident rate is more than 4.7 times greater for AD patients than elderly control subjects (Friedland 1988).

This problem is compounded by the increased severity of injuries usually sustained by older persons.

Other formidable related obstacles are encountered.

- Individuals with AD who continue to drive pose a thorny issue, largely because such mobility often represents the chief basis for independence of the patient or a spouse.
- There is gross underdeclaration in the self-reporting systems commonly used for license renewal.

- Patients with suspected dementia may refuse to surrender their licenses voluntarily. They even may claim breach of confidentiality if such suspicion were to be reported by a physician.

3

THE ISSUE OF HEREDITY

*Thus the results of modern study of heredity need not be accepted in a
form so crude that the inevitable outcome is fatalism.*

J. Arthur Thomson (1861-1933)
(British professor of natural history)

*The potentialities of tissues and consciousness actualize only through
the chemical, physical, physiological, and mental
factors of such environment. One cannot distinguish
in general, the inherited from the acquired.**

Alexis Carrel
(*Man, the Unknown* 1935)

The belief is widespread that Alzheimer's disease (AD) "runs in families." By erroneously implying predetermination to AD in the majority of cases, however, *this fatalistic attitude serves to undermine emphasis on its prevention.*

The inference that some "hereditary" factor is paramount in AD generates four important related considerations.

- *Genetic predisposition must be distinguished from "generational" exposure to neurotoxic influences among persons living in the same household.* They include a commonality of diet, habits, and exposure to a host of potentially toxic substances in the environment.

- *Heredity does not operate in a vacuum.* Stated differently, inborn metabolic or immunologic aberrations usually require an "acquired" exposure before becoming manifest. For example, hay fever might never develop if a predisposed person did not come in contact with offending pollens.

- *The inherited influence may entail altered physiology that affects the entire body rather than a disturbance solely involving the brain.* The brain becomes highly vulnerable when such a genetic aberration interferes with the availability of adequate energy, oxygen or neurotransmitters. Blass, Baker and Ko (1990) suggested that the genes contributing to AD "are expressed in extraneural tissues, although they significantly impair the function only of the cells in the clinically affected target tissue, the brain."

One likely candidate is severe hypoglycemia ("low blood and tissue sugar") due to diabetogenic hyperinsulinism (Chapter 8).

Another disorder involves the apolipoprotein E type 4 gene located within the region on chromosome 19q13.2 (Corder 1993). Its frequency has been found to be three times higher in AD patients. ApoE accumulates within the amyloid plaque and also intracellularly in neurofibrillary tangles (Chapter 4) (Poirier 1993). One-fourth of the population carries it, 2-3 percent being homozygotes. (Persons with apoE4 also are at increased risk of coronary heart disease.)

Persons with E2, an uncommon variant of apoE4, appear to be less susceptible to AD. However, Roses et al (1994) stressed that while the inheritance of one or two apoE 4/4 alleles provides a biological risk factor, it does not predict the diagnosis of AD at present because of limited epidemiological data.

- *Relatives of patients with AD should attempt to avoid as many of the risk factors and exposures enumerated in Section IV as possible.*

"Genetic" Is NOT Synonymous with "Familial"

Repeated reference to this theme is necessary. It also has been emphasized by others. The Task Force on Alzheimer's Disease of the U.S. Department of Health and Human Services (1984) indicated that "familial" is not the same as "genetic"—that is, other family members who develop AD might have been exposed at an early age to neurotoxins in the same household. Research reveals that:

- Identical and fraternal twins usually have <u>not</u> shown a tendency to develop AD—referred to as a low concordance rate. Stated differently, the concordance of AD is similar among identical and fraternal twins (Nee 1986). This implies more than one dominant gene or that nongenetic mechanisms also are operative.

- Gene linkages are relatively infrequent in other "familial" degenerative disorders of the nervous system. For example, only five to ten percent of cases of amyotrophic lateral sclerosis (Chapter 5) prove to be familial, even though the gene for this condition has been localized to chromosome 21 (Siddique 1991).

FAMILIAL DATA

The risk of developing AD is estimated to be increased as much as fourfold for persons having close relatives with this disease. Studies of some families suggest an autosomal dominant genetic pattern.

- The term "autosomal" indicates that the gene is not on a sex-linked (X or Y) chromosome.

- The term "phenotype" refers to the outward or evident makeup of an individual. It represents the product of genetic and nongenetic factors.

- A phenotype is said to be "dominant" when a single dose of a gene (that is, from one parent) causes a given effect.

The following observations are pertinent:

- In a study by the Ramsey Foundation Brain Bank (Mendez 1991), only a family history of dementia had statistical significance when compared to other aspects of the history antedating dementia.

- Breitner (1991) estimated the lifetime incidence of AD among relatives of AD patients to be 19 percent. This was three to four times the risk for relatives of control subjects.

- Persons with a first-degree relative who had AD are generally younger when AD develops (Mendez 1991). There is controversy as to whether they tend to have a more severe clinical course.

Such familial subgroups, however, have been found in less than 10-15 percent of AD cases. Admittedly, the early death of parents and grandparents ("the censoring phenomenon"), and their lack of exposure to many contemporary neurotoxins, may have lessened the percentage.

Kennedy et al (1993) compared the clinical, neuropsychological and PET imaging (Chapter 4) characteristics of 15 patients with "familial" AD, and 15 patients with "sporadic" AD. The familial cases were significantly younger, were more likely to have marked muscle spasms (myoclonus), and had preserved naming skills.

In another study of 311 AD patients, using a liberal criterion for diagnosis, Duara et al (1993) concluded that 36 percent had "familial" rather than "sporadic" AD. They noted the tendency in the familial group for an earlier age of onset, and the greater frequency of inheritance from mothers than fathers ("maternal genomic imprinting")... as occurs in Down's syndrome (mongolism). A preponderance of women also were found in the sporadic group (Chapter 16). These investigators, however, concluded that both forms represent the *same* disease.

GENE STUDIES

Most investigators seeking a specific gene from the DNA of persons with familial AD have reported "markers" on chromosome 21. This is the same chromosome involved in Down's syndrome. However, either an abnormal gene was not detected on this chromosome in some families afflicted with AD, or it involved at least two other chromosomes.

Both the early-onset form and the late-onset form of familial AD appear to be inherited as autosomal dominant traits. The early-onset form has been linked to the amyloid precursor protein (APP) gene on chromosome 21 and an unidentified gene on chromosome 14; the late-onset form is related to a gene on chromosome 19 associated with apolipoprotein E type 4 (ApoE4) (Borgaonkar 1993).

The phenomenon of *genetic heterogeneity* poses another consideration in AD. This refers to a similar clinical pattern (phenotype) in persons with different genotypes… as from three or more separate locations of the gene (Breitner 1991). A case in point is variation of the beta-amyloid precursor protein (APP) gene (Chapter 4) in AD patients from diverse population groups (United States, England, Japan, France).

Murrell et al (1991) provided important evidence that mutation involving a single amino acid may be operative in AD. They studied a family with classic early-onset, autopsy-proven AD in which an autosomal dominant inheritance pattern appeared to affect three generations. Direct sequencing of DNA revealed substitution of phenylalanine (Chapters 7 and 9) for valine in the transmembrane domain of the amyloid precursor protein—specifically at position 1924.

4

BRAIN CHANGES

*We must turn to nature itself, to the observations of the body
in health and disease, to learn the truth.*

Hippocrates

*Disease is very old and nothing about it has changed.
It is we who change as we learn to recognize what
was formerly imperceptible.*

Dr. J. M. Charcot
(19th Century neurologist)

Several characteristic changes occur in the brain of patients with Alzheimer's disease (AD). Indeed, this diagnosis only can be made with certainty by demonstrating these findings at autopsy or in tissue obtained by biopsy. Some clinicians therefore prefer the term "probable Alzheimer's disease" (Chapter 1).

A brief review of the pathologic changes is presented here because terms such as senile plaques and neurofibrillary tangles will be mentioned repeatedly. Since most readers of this book are not health professionals, medical terms will be minimized. Further details can be found in most neurology and pathology texts, and in the references provided.

INTRODUCTORY PERSPECTIVES

This chapter is prefaced with a basic premise: *Alzheimer's disease probably represents a chronic reaction of the brain to multiple adverse influences to which the general population is subjected, with or without a genetic predisposition.* The nature of such exposures and the supporting evidences will be presented in subsequent chapters—with emphasis on disturbed metabolism and environmental neurotoxins.

This perspective is consistent with the suspicion of Alzheimer (1907) himself. Deducing that the observed "peculiar substance" resulted from metabolic changes, he wrote: "The conversion of the fibril seems to go hand in hand with the storage of a pathologic metabolic product in the ganglion cell, a possibility which needs to be more deeply researched."

Neuropathologists recognize that other neuropathologic processes can occur in the AD patient. This is most evident in "mixed dementia" resulting from both AD and cerebrovascular disease.

BRAIN SIZE

Patients diagnosed as having AD may or may not evidence <u>decreased brain size</u> by computerized tomography (CT) or magnetic resonance imaging (MRI). When present, changes in brain volume can be quantified by MRI, both in its entirety and in an area crucial to memory known as the hippocampus. This structure is uniquely vulnerable to insults caused by decreased nutrition (Chapters 7 and 8), neurotoxins (Chapters 9-11), and lack of oxygen (Chapter 12).

Many investigators (Kesslak 1991, Scheltens 1991a, Jack 1992, Pasquier 1994) have confirmed that there is significant shrinking or atrophy of the hippocampus in AD (Figure 4-1).

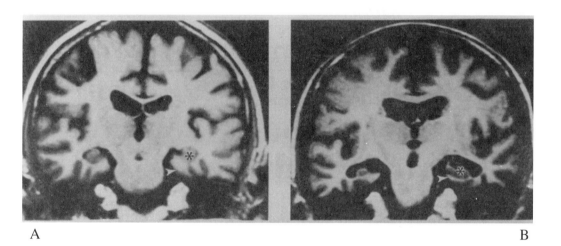

A   B

Figure 4-1

Kesslak, J.P., Nalcioglu, O., Cotman, C.W.
Quantification of magnetic resonance scans for hippocampal and
    parahippocampal atrophy in Alzheimer's disease.
Neurology 1991; 41:51-54. (© 1991 *Neurology.* Reproduced with
    permission)

MRI image of a control subject (A) showing an intact and well-formed
hippocampus (*) and parahippocampal gyrus (arrow). The AD patient
(B) evidences a significant reduction in the volume of these structures as
well as diffuse atrophy of the cerebral cortex "gray matter."

- Kesslak et al (1991) correlated such atrophy with severity of the dementia (Scheltens 1991) and Mini-Mental State Examination scores (Chapter 1).

- Pasquier (1994) suggested that medial temporal lobe atrophy noted by CT studies is an effective test for AD among persons below the age of 70, even in its early clinical stages.

Jobst (1994) reported that atrophy of the medial temporal lobe averages 15.1 percent per year in patients with confirmed AD, compared to 1.5 percent in healthy aging controls. They regarded this phenomenon as vulnerability of the medial temporal lobe to various stresses—with the probable initiation of a pathological cascade process—and not acceleration of normal age-related atrophy. This perspective underscores the need for identifying such pathophysiologic triggers, and the possible prevention of AD by protecting vulnerable neurons.

These observations have clinical relevance.

- Baulac et al (1993) found atrophy of the hippocampus and another structure, the amygdala, to be significant even in "mild" stages of AD. This enabled separating such patients from controls.

- de Leon et al (1993) regard hippocampal atrophy as a biological marker that precedes AD symptoms. They conducted a four-year longitudinal study of non-demented elderly individuals. The baseline data could predict dementia with sensitivities and specificities of about 90 percent—including correlations for delayed memory recall.

- There is increasing evidence for the practical usefulness of single-photon emission computed tomography (SPECT) as a diagnostic modality in patients suspected of having mild AD (Claus 1994). Decreased cerebral blood flow to the temporal region appears to be the best discriminating variable between patients and controls, especially with greater severity of the dementia.

BRAIN PHYSIOLOGY

Long ago, Hippocrates related disturbed behavior to structural changes within specific areas of the brain—most notably in his book on epilepsy, *The Sacred Disease*.

The validation of this concept is strikingly evidenced in AD by the characteristic pattern of changes involving regional brain blood flow, glucose metabolism, and oxygen utilization in the brain noted by positron emission tomography (PET). The changes usually involve the parietal lobes in a relatively symmetrical fashion, possibly with extension into the adjacent temporal and occipital lobes.

MICROSCOPIC FINDINGS

The characteristic findings in AD are amyloid (senile) plaques, neurofibrillary tangles (NFTs), and loss of nerve cells (neurons) and nerve synapses (connections). Since they might be detected in patients with other neurologic disorders who may or may not have clinical dementia (Chapter 15), common underlying mechanisms are probably operative.

Amyloid (Senile) Plaques (Figure 4-2)

A definitive diagnosis of AD <u>requires</u> the demonstration of many amyloid plaques. These spherical structures have a central core of beta-amyloid (see below) from which distended nerve endings (neurites) radiate. Although their distribution in localized areas is less rigidly defined than for NFTs, the number of senile plaques tends to correlate with the degree of dementia.

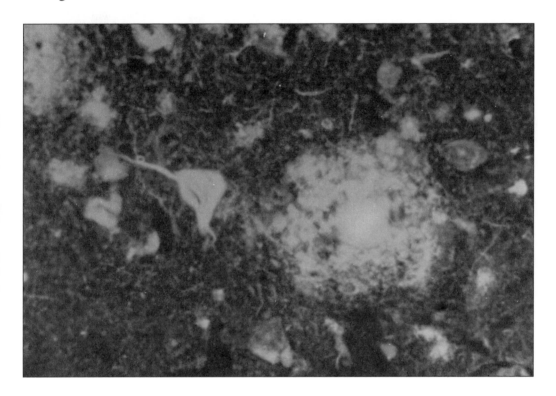

Figure 4-2

A microscopic image of two senile plaques and a large neurofibrillary tangle. One plaque is in the corner; the other, with a prominent central core, occupies the center of the field. The tangle lies within a neuron between the two plaques. A normal neuron without abnormal fibers is present on the opposite side of the center plaque. (Courtesy of Robert Terry, M.D.)

Neurofibrillary Tangles (Figure 4-2)

NFTs are <u>not</u> specific for AD, in contrast to the deposition of many amyloid plaques. These twisted nerve endings have been likened to tennis rackets or pretzels. They are chiefly found in the cerebral cortex ("gray matter") and the hippocampus. The presence of large numbers has correlated with the severity of dementia (Arriagada 1992).

Neurofibrillary tangles represent "cellular tombstones" of dead nerve cells. These

37

insoluble masses of paired helical elements, composed of abnormal tau proteins, impair cellular function and slow neurotransmission. Their consistent localization to specific layers of the hippocampus and cerebral cortex (Hyman 1991a) is probably influenced by the unique metabolic characteristics of such areas (Chapter 8).

These findings also are noteworthy:

- NFTs tend to form <u>early</u> during the disease. They accumulate in so-called association areas of the brain as dementia progresses (Arriagada 1991).

- *There is a lapse of 20 to 30 years between development of the first tangles and the marked pathologic changes associated with cognitive failure* (Hyman 1990, 1991).

- Tangles have been detected in the brains of <u>nondemented</u> persons over the age of 55 (Hyman 1990). This suggests the likelihood that AD would have developed had they lived longer.

- Analysis of the distribution of Alzheimer-type pathologic changes in nondemented elderly individuals matches the pattern in AD (Arriagada 1992).

- *The comparable distribution of pathologic findings in both demented and nondemented older persons is consistent with the concept of a continuum between elderly nondemented individuals, persons with "early" or evolving AD, and the full-blown disease* (Chapter 6).

Payan et al (1992) made another important observation. They reported that proteins associated with NFTs contain a significantly greater number of two modified amino acid (aspartyl) residues than unaffected proteins from the surrounding gray matter or comparable preparations from normal brain. Schapira and Chou (1987) also reported excess D-aspartate in NFTs and senile plaques. The significance of these amino acid stereoisomers will be discussed in Chapters 7 and 9.

Specifically, the normal protein-bound L-aspartyl/L-asparaginyl residues change into the D-aspartate or the L-isoaspartyl forms. Twice as much defective aspartate—chiefly beta-linked L-isoaspartate—is present in NFTs than in the surrounding gray matter, and 1.5 times more than in normal brain controls.

Loss of Brain Cells and Nerve Synapses

A significant loss of cells occurs in both the cerebral cortex and certain subcortical centers of the AD brain (Figure 4-1). These centers constitute the major suppliers of neurotransmitters to higher cortical centers—including acetylcholine, norepinephrine and serotonin (Chapter 5).

The loss of nerve synapses correlates most closely with the extent of cognitive impairment. Indeed, Terry et al (1991) suggested that synapse loss represents an event more primary in AD than the accumulation of amyloid.

Deposits of Amyloid in the Brain and Blood Vessels

This degenerative change is also designated as amyloidosis of the brain and amyloid angiopathy. The disorganized plaque (see above), consisting of disintegrating fragments of brain cells and tissue, surrounds a core of hard substance called beta-amyloid outside the cells. This core consists largely of inorganic aluminosilicate (Chapter 10) and a protein (Candy 1986). The latter is derived from precursor proteins collectively referred to as amyloid precursor protein (APP).

> Although the term means starch-like, it is a unique protein now called *beta-amyloid*. Murphy (1992) reviewed the nature of this protein and its *amyloid precursor protein* (APP).

Beta-amyloid is formed from APP by protein-degrading machinery that exists in healthy cells. It therefore has a normal function, presumably to protect neurons against biophysiologic dangers (lack of glucose and oxygen), neurotoxic exposure, and physical injury—perhaps through preventing the accumulation of excessive calcium. For example, deposits of beta-amyloid have been noted in human brain several days after head trauma (Roberts 1991).

> The normal neuroprotective role of APP peptides has been shown by the protection of neurons against hypoglycemic damage in hippocampal cell cultures (Mattson 1993). Conversely, aberrant processing of APP can result in neurodegeneration by impairment of this neuroprotective function.

Beta-amyloid is initially deposited in the brain as diffuse plaques. But over the years, other proteins and supportive (glial) cells become embedded, perhaps in part reflecting an immune response.

Considerable beta-amyloid may become neurotoxic, especially when it accumulates in cells (Marx 1992). It has both a direct neurotoxic effect and an indirect one—that is, by making neurons more vulnerable to excitotoxic insults.

- Mattson et al (1993) demonstrated that exposure of cultured human cortical neurons to beta-amyloid peptides destabilizes calcium metabolism.

- There is other experimental evidence that beta-amyloid is directly toxic to hippocampal neurons in culture (Harrigan 1993).

- Beta-amyloid increases the toxicity of various excitotoxins such as glutamate (Chapter 9) and calcium. One of the mechanisms is opening "holes" in the membranes of brain cells, thereby allowing the entry of excessive calcium.

There is considerable interest in the underlying role of apolipoprotein E (ApoE) type 4 allele, a relatively common gene (Corder 1993, Waldholz 1993), and the absence of E3. (At least three different genes [E2, E3, E4] exist. These have been studied as risk factors for coronary heart disease.) This cholesterol-transporting protein has a unique affinity for beta-amyloid, which it presumably can deposit in the brain. The finding that E3 tacks itself to tau at the same region as does phosphate provides also suggests the primacy of disturbed metabolism in AD.

The primary metabolic and neurotoxic changes that cause AD probably induce deterioration of nerve cells and membranes, with ensuing plaques and NFTs. Amyloid formation subsequently occurs when the usually-protected amyloid precursor protein becomes exposed, and undergoes proteolytic cleavage. If the amyloid precursor is cleaved out, amyloid tends to be deposited around cells and blood vessels

5

NEUROTRANSMITTER DYSFUNCTION

*The study of causes of things must be preceded
by the study of things caused.*

Dr. Hughlings Jackson
(A pioneer neurologist)

*As a clinical researcher, I'd be looking
for anything better than nothing.*

Trey Sunderland (1991)
(Chief of Geriatric Psychopharmacology, National Institute of Mental Health)

Neurotransmitters and related neuropeptides are chemical mediators crucial for proper function of the brain, peripheral nerves and endocrine glands. They include acetylcholine, norepinephrine, dopamine, serotonin and nerve growth factor. Because neurotransmitter dysfunction in Alzheimer's disease (AD) centers largely on acetylcholine (cholinergic effects) and nerve growth factor activity, this brief review will be limited largely to them.

Considerable current pharmacologic research in AD focuses on replacing or enhancing the depletion of neurotransmitters. Unfortunately, most drugs in this category have proved ineffective once the condition has deteriorated to the degree of being diagnosable clinically. This poses yet another reason to emphasize awareness of "early" or "evolving" AD, at which stage such therapeutic intervention might be more effective.

A basic premise of my integrated hypothesis (Chapter 6) avers that *many of the adverse metabolic, hypoxemic and neurotoxic influences operative in AD damage acetylcholine and nerve growth factor mechanisms, culminating in the depletion of these vital substances.*

40

THE CHOLINERGIC SYSTEM

The cholinergic system encompasses brain cells in the cerebral cortex ("gray matter"), the hippocampus (Chapter 4), and the basal forebrain. The basal nucleus of Meynert (nucleus basalis) constitutes a major source of cholinergic innervation and acetylcholine release (Agid 1991a).

Figure 5-1 schematically depicts the transport of acetylcholine (ACh) from the basal nucleus to nerve cells or neurons in the cerebral cortex.

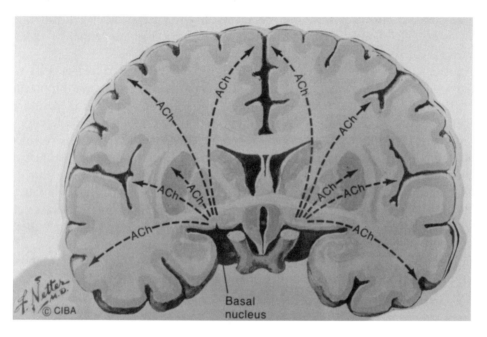

Figure 5-1

Schematic section of brain showing the normal transport of acetylcholine (ACh) from the basal nucleus of Meynert (substantia innominata) to cortical gray matter. Cholinergic nerve fibers within the basal nucleus are massively depleted in Alzheimer's disease.

ACETYLCHOLINE

The centrality of acetylcholine for nerve transmission is detailed in physiology and pharmacology texts. Its synthesis from choline and acetylcoenzyme A involves the enzyme choline acetyltransferase. In the absence of ingested choline, the choline used for synthesizing large amounts of acetylcholine probably comes from a reservoir of phosphatidylcholine in nerve membranes, a process termed "autocannibalism" (Wurtman 1990).

The enzyme acetylcholinesterase (cholinesterase; acetylcholine hydrolase; AChE) terminates nerve impulse transmission at cholinergic junctions (synapses) by rapidly transforming (hydrolyzing) acetylcholine.

Relationship of Acetylcholine to Glucose and Oxygen

The brain's mandatory requirements for an adequate and continuous supply of glucose ("body sugar") and oxygen are discussed in Chapters 8 and 12. Glucose is needed for the synthesis of acetylcholine (Quastel 1936, Brenner 1942). Furthermore, a normal glucose concentration restrains the synthesis and release of acetylcholine. These processes become stimulated at low blood glucose levels (hypoglycemia). If excessive, convulsions can result (Feldberg 1945).

Another vicious cycle may ensue. Damage to the basal forebrain caused by severe reduction of glucose also lessens glucose utilization by the cortex and hippocampus (Harrell 1985). Indeed, some investigators concluded that AD is primarily a degenerative nerve cell disorder in which a targeted loss of neocortical cholinergic neurons results from the limitation of energy. This is technically described as "a selective reduction in all glycolytic enzymes involved in hexosemonophosphate metabolism" (Bowen 1979).

Malnutrition contributes to the problem, especially during the periods of infancy and childhood (Chapters 7 and 8). In experimental studies, total brain cholinesterase activity is low in newborn rats subjected to protein malnutrition, and remains so even after providing a normal diet (Im 1971).

Dramatic changes in acetylcholine concentrations also occur during and after reduced blood supply (ischemia) to the brain, with an associated decrease of transport oxygen (Chapter 12).

Cholinergic Depletion in Alzheimer's Disease

A massive depletion—up to 90 percent—of cholinergic fibers has been found within the basal nucleus in AD. By contrast, there is relative sparing of other neurotransmitters (dopamine; gamma-aminobutyric acid; somatostatin) in the brain of AD patients.

The production of beta-amyloid (Chapter 4) appears to be accelerated by reduced levels of acetylcholine (Wurtman 1993).

Pathology within these forebrain neurons, which also express nerve growth factor activity (see below), results in cholinergic dysfunction. (This is referred to as "cholinergic deafferentation of telencephalic targets.") A reduction or loss of various cholinergic markers, such as the enzyme choline acetyltransferase, has been demonstrated in areas of cholinergic innervation within the AD brain (Kerwin 1991). This may occur as well during transitional AD—that is, before overt dementia (Zweig 1989). The dementia, however, cannot be attributed solely to modest depletion of acetylcholine.

> Scopolamine, an anticholinergic drug, can induce transient cognitive deficits in normal older persons, but does not alter attention or fluency (Ownby 1991). Moreover, it increases brain metabolism in such individuals... contrasting with the decreased regional brain metabolism that characterizes AD (Ownby 1991) (Chapter 8).

Cholinesterase Activity in Alzheimer's Disease

The extent of cholinergic dysfunction in AD is indicated by cholinesterase-positive activity within at least three-fourths of the amyloid plaques and neurofibrillary tangles (Mesulam 1987). Mesulam et al (1991) subsequently demonstrated cholinesterase activity at all three sites of abnormal protein deposition in AD—namely, the plaques, tangles, and amyloid angiopathy (Chapter 4). (The cortical vessels of AD patients without amyloid angiopathy are generally free of cholinesterase activity.) These observations suggest the synthesis of cholinesterase-like substances by the remaining cholinergic neurons in response to underlying metabolic derangements.

NERVE GROWTH FACTOR

The various metabolic abnormalities and neurotoxic exposures conducive to AD can alter and deplete nerve growth factor (NGF). The ensuing interruption of metabolic or trophic support may cause or contribute to nerve cell death.

Information concerning NGF and its receptor has exploded within the past decade. NGF is known to be critical for the survival of certain groups of nerve cells known as ganglia during development of the nervous system.

- NGF stimulates the sprouting of projections through which neurons contact one another.

- NGF supports the long-term survival of nondividing neurons.

- NGF can induce choline acetyltransferase activity, and promote the growth and survival of basal forebrain cholinergic neurons (Fischer 1987).

Nerve growth factor and related substances—basic fibroblast growth factor (bFGF), and insulin-like growth factors (IGF-I and IGF-II)—can protect hippocampal and septal neurons against damage caused by hypoglycemia. Such neuroprotection is indicated by the ability of neuronal mitochondria to accumulate the fluorescent dye rhodamine-123 (Mattson 1993) (Chapter 8).

Relationship to Glucose

There are pertinent interrelations between NGF and glucose metabolism.

- Both NGF and insulin are structurally, functionally and evolutionarily related proteins (Frazier 1973).

- NGF affects glucose metabolism of the sympathetic and sensory nerve cells (Angeletti 1964).

- The addition of NGF markedly increases the oxidation of glucose to carbon dioxide—probably by activating the hexosemonophosphate pathway in nerve cells.

An interesting relationship between diabetes mellitus and abnormal NGF metabolism is the increase of "NGF receptor-truncated" in the urine of patients with diabetic neuropathy (Hruska 1993). This soluble cleavage product of the NGF-receptor also is elevated in plasma and urine after nerve injury (such as section of the sciatic nerve) and in patients with amyotrophic lateral sclerosis (ALS).

Nerve Growth Factor in Alzheimer's Disease

The underlying metabolic and/or toxicologic injury causing AD probably severely depletes brain acetylcholine (see above) through the degeneration of NGF-responsive neurons in the basal forebrain. This cholinergic loss appears to be secondary to NGF depletion (Yankner 1991a). The mechanisms might involve altered synthesis or transport of NGF for its trophic support of neurons in the cortex and hippocampus. For example, neurofibrillary tangles could interfere with the delivery of NGF to their neurons.

The following observations are pertinent:

- An overall reduction in NGF-receptor axons and terminals has been reported both in AD and old age (Kerwin 1991).

- There is evidence for selective vulnerability of those neurons that express NGF receptor (Agid 1991b). Moreover, the changes therein appear to precede a loss of cholinergic neurons.

- NGF can ameliorate both age-related and lesion-induced degeneration of cholinergic neurons in adult animals (Tuszynski 1991).

- Rabizadeh et al (1993) demonstrated the binding or locking of NGF to a low-affinity NGF receptor (p75[NGFR]). This is required for survival of those nerve cells in the nucleus basalis of Meynert that are destroyed in AD. The existence of such binding provides potential clues to its prevention and treatment.

OTHER NEUROTRANSMITTERS

Disturbances involving additional neuropeptides probably play a role in the causation of AD (Khachaturian 1989). The depletion of such neurotransmitters in AD, especially norepinephrine and serotonin, may have clinical expressions.

- A reduction of cells containing norepinephrine has been reported in the locus ceruleus of AD patients (Harik 1991). This structure is critical for proper function of the brain's norepinephrine nerve pathways.

- The occurrence of narcolepsy (pathologic drowsiness and sleep) in AD patients (Chapter 15) can be explained in part by the depletion of norepinephrine-containing cells (Roberts 1971b).

- Deficits of serotonin in the AD brain (Bowen 1990) may be manifest clinically as sleep abnormalities and psychiatric features.

SECTION II

THE CAUSATION OF ALZHEIMER'S DISEASE

*We know what causes AIDS. We have no idea
what causes Alzheimer's Disease.*

Bentley Lipscomb (1991)
(Director, Florida Department of Elder Affairs)

*Even when each of these areas is considered in isolation, one
is led to the conclusion that AD is not a single entity
but rather can arise from multiple causes.*

M. P. Mattson et al (1993)

*In light of what is known about Alzheimer's disease, is there
some way of drawing all these divergent observations into a
cohesive theory about how Alzheimer's disease actually
damages the brain?… This would mean that the
medical community is not faced with
identifying and treating one condition,
but several conditions.**

S. L. Shalat (1989)

6

THE EVOLUTION OF ALZHEIMER'S DISEASE: AN INTEGRATED HYPOTHESIS

Observe patiently, experiment cautiously, and generalize slowly.

Bacon

A theory is the more impressive the greater is the simplicity of its premises, the more different are the kinds of things it relates, and the more extended is its range of applicability.

Albert Einstein

The invention of other new theories regularly and appropriately evokes the same response from some of these specialists on whose area of special competence they impinge. For these men the new theory implies a change in the rules governing the prior practice of normal science. *

Thomas S. Kuhn (1970)

Any theory about the nature of Alzheimer's disease (AD) also must account for its emergence and progression as an epidemic during this century (Chapter 2). The following panoramic hypothesis satisfies this requirement. It is based on extensive personal observations, published researches concerning pertinent metabolic, neurologic and toxicologic disorders, and the findings of other investigators.

- *Alzheimer's disease represents a type of response by the brain to injury resulting from altered nutrition and metabolism, multiple exogenous neurotoxins in food, water, air and drugs, deficient oxygen (hypoxemia), and other forms of stress.*

- *Physiological, dietary, technological and societal influences—with or without specific genetic vulnerability—can initiate the characteristic brain changes.*

- *Such damage tends to be compounded over time by trauma, altered circulation to the brain, and immunologic reactions resulting from exposure to toxic chemicals and even public health interventions (e.g., multiple immunizations).*

- *These adverse effects ultimately culminate in a significant loss of vital nerve cells (neurons) within the highly integrated memory neurosystem that are unable to regenerate.*

- *The same noxious influences contribute to degenerative* changes elsewhere in the nervous system as well as other vulnerable organs—for example, the peripheral nerves, lens, retina and inner ear.*

General Commentary

Conclusions independently drawn by others validate this concept. Discussing the Framingham Study of AD patients, Bachman et al (1992) stated: "Dementia… is not a single disease but is the end result of a number of disease processes that may occur separately or together in any one individual."

The foregoing theory also is consistent with the evolving belief that cell-death pathways or apoptosis (from the Greek word meaning "a falling off") are inappropriately activated in AD and other neurodegenerative diseases (Shaffer 1993).

PRIMARY FACTORS

The following adverse factors appear to play a primary role in both initiating AD, and driving its progression. (They are not necessarily listed according to their importance or sequence.) Each will be addressed in subsequent chapters.

I. Recurrent depletion of energy (substrate) within highly vulnerable areas of the brain

The brain is virtually totally dependent on the delivery of an adequate and continuous supply of glucose or "body sugar." Any decrease in the amount of circulating glucose to brain tissue—referred to as cerebral glucopenia—can be highly damaging, especially during childhood and early adult life.

II. Secretion of excessive insulin by persons subject to reactive hypoglycemia ("low blood sugar attacks"), with ensuing deprivation of glucose for the brain

This *frequent* disorder is also termed "functional" hyperinsulinism and "diabetogenic" hyperinsulinism.

III. Increased production and/or release of insulin in various ways, thereby exaggerating cerebral glucopenia

These factors include ingesting excessive sugar, protein and calories, contemporary eating habits, and aging.

---

*The term "degenerative" refers to the shriveling and disappearance of cells in the absence of inflammation or an interruption of their blood supply.

IV. <u>Adverse metabolic and toxic effects on vital brain cells and other tissues caused by</u> <u>unprecedented technologic innovations</u>

Particular emphasis is placed on highly processed foods, food additives, and numerous chemicals in air, water, food and drugs. They may result in direct neuronal injury, or the depletion of important neurotransmitters and nerve growth factors (Chapter 5) needed for proper nerve and brain function.

ADDITIONAL MAJOR FACTORS

The following influences also can cause or aggravate disordered brain function.

- <u>Reduced oxygen to the brain</u> (Chapter 12). A reduction in oxygen supply may result from smoking, exposure to carbon monoxide (vehicles; certain occupations), air travel, high altitudes, and vascular changes involving blood vessels in the brain and neck.

- <u>The effects of aluminum</u> (Chapter 10). The mechanisms include direct aluminum toxicity, changes in the blood-brain barrier, and altered metabolism.

- <u>The effects of many drugs</u> (Chapter 12). The offending drugs include common psychoactive agents (sedatives; tranquilizers) and anesthetics.

- <u>Novel food products and certain food additives containing large amounts of</u> <u>single amino acids that can cross the blood-brain barrier, and alter vital</u> <u>neurotransmitter function at nerve membranes</u> (Chapters 7 and 9).

- <u>The increased vulnerability of many unsuspected "carriers" (heterozygotes) for</u> <u>several major hereditary disorders (Chapter 14) to potential dietary neurotoxins.</u>

- <u>"Radiation stress" from artificial lighting sources</u> (Chapter 16).

- <u>Chronic psychologic stress</u> (Chapter 13).

- <u>Chronic behavioral stress—including the effects of dramatic changes in work</u> <u>habits, time shifts, and information overload</u> (Chapter 13).

- <u>Various responses of the immune system.</u> Immunologic (autoimmune) mechanisms have been invoked in the causation of other degenerative nervous system disorders, especially multiple sclerosis, amyotrophic lateral sclerosis and myasthenia gravis. They might play a role in amyloid formation (Chapter 4) and altered acetylcholine metabolism (Chapter 5). There is some evidence for a role of localized inflammatory reaction in AD—including the presence of acute phase reactants in plaques, and the ability of amyloid to activate complement.

  The immunologic component of AD has been stressed by Dr. H. Hugh Fudenberg (1993), an immune system researcher. He underscores the role of so-called transfer factor, a natural compound obtained from helper T-lymphocytes that accept hormones and releasing factors from the hypothalamus. Other lymphocytes and monocytes (resembling microglial cells in the brain) are involved with neurotransmitter function (Chapter 5) and the disposal of foreign material.

THE CONCEPT OF TRANSITIONAL ALZHEIMER'S DISEASE

In order to understand AD and institute measures aimed at its prevention, I shall emphasize the importance of certain clinical, physiologic and tissue changes (pathology) during its *"evolving"* or *"transitional"* phase. This refers to the period *before* overt dementia resulting from excessive and irreversible brain damage. Beyreuther et al (1991) estimated that this period, during which beta-amyloid (Chapter 4) accumulates, lasts 30 years! Other synonyms I shall use include *"early AD"* and *"the AD-prone state."*

Such a prolonged hiatus is consistent with many of the demographic, clinical and pathological observations about AD cited in other chapters. As a corollary to attempted prevention, physicians must "THINK ALZHEIMER'S!" when confronted with unexplained neuropsychiatric features in patients who do not yet display gross memory loss. Some examples include "benign positional vertigo" and "chronic fatigue" (Chapters 15 and 16).

- Hachinski (1992) referred to a symptomless "brain-at-risk" stage in which symptoms or signs may not be present.

- Slight focal impairment of cognition in the warning "pre-dementia" stage, coupled with marked hippocampal atrophy (Chapter 4), should alert the clinician to "early" AD.

- The finding of neurofibrillary tangles as "early pathologic changes" in an area of the brain known the limbic cortex (Chapter 4), and their accumulation in the brain's "association areas" with progression of dementia (Hyman 1991, Arriagada 1991), validate the prolonged evolutionary phase.

- Morris et al (1991) found <u>marked</u> changes in the brains of 10 patients with "very mild Alzheimer's disease."

In prior researches, I sought risk factors during the evolution of other diseases. They included "transitional" multiple sclerosis (Roberts 1966b,c), proneness to traffic accidents (Roberts 1971b), and pre-thrombotic ischemic (coronary) heart disease (Roberts 1967a, 1991b). It is now universally accepted that attention to risk factors for coronary heart disease constitutes a cornerstone in preventing heart attacks.

This concept of a transitional phase also clarifies the <u>overlap or continuum</u> of brain changes noted in "aging" as well as AD. It is consistent with the existence of a considerable reserve of neurons, and extraordinary attempts by the brain to compensate for cell damage resulting from energy depletion and exposure to neurotoxins. The "error theory" of aging avers that an accumulation of random damage caused by many possible events activates an "age" gene.

- Noting that the distribution of Alzheimer-type changes in <u>nondemented</u> elderly individuals matches that found in AD, Arriagada et al (1992) stated: "The observation of a consistent anatomic distribution of the pathologic findings across all the cases, and its similarity to that seen in AD, favors a continuum in the pathologic process between elderly nondemented individuals, those with early preclinical stages of AD, and AD."

- Brayne and Calloway (1988) suggested that normal aging, "benign senescent forgetfulness," and senile dementia of the Alzheimer type (SDAT) represent the continuum of a common underlying process.

It is necessary to distinguish the basic cause(s) of AD (e.g., numerous potential neurotoxins in the environment) from mechanisms that contribute to its clinical and pathologic expressions. Insights about the latter continue to emerge from many laboratories. For example, the prominent "resprouting" of nerve cells apparently represents a compensatory phenomenon by the surviving neurons to fill gaps left by dead neurons, assisted by the production of amyloid precursor protein (APP) (Chapter 4). The excessive production of APP is probably initiated by prior neurotoxic influences.

COMMENTARY ON ORIGINS OF THE HYPOTHESIS
AND ANTICIPATED CRITICISM

Origins

My role as a primary-care physician, who has personally followed the course of many patients over decades *before* they evidenced a dementing illness, afforded the extraordinary opportunity to crystallize these concepts. I have been able to analyze the detailed records of such patients for common clues that might provide comprehensible "risk factors" for AD. This approach is consistent with the age-old challenge: "Seek, and ye shall find" (*Matthew 7:7*).

Few neurologists have the benefit of comparable prolonged first-hand contact with patients when they were relatively well neurologically. But more than simple observation is required. Charles Gow aptly commented: "Observation is more than seeing; it is knowing what you see and comprehending its significance."

To propose some specific "cause" for AD is inherently misleading in most instances. For example, it is probably incorrect to postulate a *single* genetic mechanism that *unilaterally* predestines brain cell destruction (Chapter 3). Rather, its causation appears to be multifactorial and cumulative over time. The initial insult in a given individual—whether metabolic, neurotoxic or traumatic—might represent a "chaotic" event. (Such a generality has been invoked for many aspects of evolution.) The truism that any major action in nature evokes a comparable reaction seems equally appropriate.

The element of serendipity (fortunate chance) also contributed to my interest in AD. It had been kindled over three decades during seemingly unrelated research projects involving narcolepsy, migraine, reading disability, seizures, multiple sclerosis, diabetic neuropathy, other neurologic disorders, and reactions to products containing aspartame (NutraSweet®).

Criticism

I endorse the need for considerable skepticism and intense scrutiny of any theory—including mine—that purports to explain the causation of AD. However, critical peers who challenge the foregoing hard-earned insights must be prepared to demonstrate and justify in detail perceived major errors or deficiencies of my panoramic hypothesis. This is important for two reasons. First, the hypothesis appears to provide a rational approach for the prevention of AD. Second, it offers constructive suggestions about *reasonable* measures that might prevent or retard further neurologic deterioration during the suspected "transitional" phase of this disease.

Dr. William Landau stressed the theme of "clinical neuroskepticism" relative to neurologic disorders in an address to the annual meeting of the American Academy of Neurology (April 28, 1993). He recalled the statement by Thomas Jefferson in 1782: "Ignorance is preferable to error." As an example, he critically reviewed the so-called carotid sinus syndrome in the context of often having been a misnomer for transient cerebral ischemic attacks.

"Authorities" who have close corporate associations (e.g., as employees, consultants or recipients of research funding) should restrain dogmatic denials of neurotoxic hazards that could be interpreted as serving corporate interests. Such bias also risks accusations of scientific "shills" or "sellouts" (Dukes 1993).

I have encountered this type of unyielding criticism in the case of adverse reactions to pentachlorophenol (Roberts 1990), excessive vitamin E intake (Roberts 1981c, 1984b), antistatic clothes softeners (Roberts 1986), and products containing aspartame (Roberts 1987b, 1988c, 1989a, 1992b). The same phenomenon also exists in other spheres.

- "Truth squads" of urologists vigorously denied my repeated warnings over three decades about the potential increased risks of cancer and autoimmune disorders in young men after contraceptive vasectomy (Roberts 1979, 1993). Recent studies, both prospective and retrospective, have confirmed a striking increase of prostate cancer in such men, especially 20 years or more postoperatively (Giovannucci 1993a,b).

- "Experts" residing in protected environments reflexively deny the complaints by farm laborers of severe solar skin irritation that predictably occurs after rocket launches—perhaps reflecting transient greater depletion of the protective ozone layer.

7

THE ROLE OF DIET AND NUTRITION

Whatsoever is the father of disease, an ill diet was its mother.

George Herbert

*The [food] issue is a larger one than is realized by the public.
The practice reflects what is happening to our entire food
supply, namely a lowering of food quality which
results in nutritional shortchanging.**

Beatrice Trum Hunter (1977)

*The rights of physicians and patients are recklessly violated
by frauds in foods and drugs... The subject of food ethics is
one of the most important of all that come before this
Section in my opinion.*

Dr. Efraim Cutter (1893)

Extraordinary changes in nutrition during the 20th Century probably have contributed to the escalation of Alzheimer's disease (AD). They encompass excessive intake of calories, sugar and protein; radical changes in eating habits; innovations in food technology and preparation; greater access to these products; and the ravages of malnutrition (voluntary or imposed) early in life.

The progressive depletion of soils is also relevant. Fruits and vegetables purchased in most markets tend to have decreased micronutrients. Smith (1993) compared the amount in pears, apples, sweet corn and potatoes grown in the conventional way and by "organic" gardening. Selenium, manganese, sodium, magnesium, strontium, potassium

---

*Reproduced with permission of Beatrice Trum Hunter.

and lithium were increased in the organically-grown products. Conversely, the organic foods contained less aluminum, lead, mercury and cadmium.

Others have expressed comparable concern in more generalized terms.

- Sir William Osler issued this warning about culinary adventurism: "Cookery simulates the disguise of medicine and pretends to know what food is best for the body."

- Beatrice Trum Hunter (1977) noted that "… traditional foods have undergone radical transformations in processing. Every untried and untested change is fraught with possibilities of adverse effect on human health."

- The harmonious relationship between the earth and living creatures was recognized centuries ago by American Indians. Chief Seattle observed: "The earth does not belong to man. Man belongs to the earth."

- There have been various versions of the statement by Jean Anthelme Brillat-Savarin, an 19th Century gastronome: "Tell me what you eat, and I'll tell you what you are."

- Another Frenchman asserted: "The better you eat, the better you will think."

Contributory Factors and Habits

The following phenomena are noteworthy. They will be amplified both in the following discussion and subsequent chapters.

- De-emphasis of breast-feeding and increased reliance on the substitution of artificial infant formulas

- Prolonged overnight fasting, especially among young children and older persons

- Missed meals, coupled with "forced feeding"—i.e., eating only one or two meals a day

- Hurried eating—"wolfing down" food or "eating on the run"—which is conducive to the "dumping phenomenon" that results in excessive wasting of insulin and hypoglycemia (Chapter 8)

- Excessive sugar consumption

- Excessive protein consumption

- Chemical and physical modification of oils by hydrogenation—a process favored by processors because such oils, when heated, do not smoke readily, can be used for quick deep-fat frying, and are less likely to turn rancid

- Excessive caffeine intake from coffee, tea and cola drinks

- The introduction of many novel foodstuffs and individual amino acids that are potentially neurotoxic, especially to carriers of some common metabolic diseases

- Increased exposure to mirror images (stereoisomers) of amino acids, sugars and fats resulting from overheating, prolonged storage, and technologic manipulations

- Excessive iron in "fortified" food products (Chapter 9)

- The widespread use of potentially neurotoxic additives, especially aspartame and monosodium glutamate (MSG) (Chapter 9)

Other Innovations in Food Technology

Techniques that lengthen the shelf life of products or give foods an improved appearance also must be considered. They include thousands of food chemicals and dyes, such as sulfiting agents, the nitrites, and the synthetic butylated antioxidants (BHA/BHT).

"Active packaging" is another innovation. It involves incorporating metallic heat susceptors in plastic food packaging intended for microwave cooking (Hunter 1991b).

Hunter (1993) reviewed a number of unanticipated interactions involving other plastic materials.

- Volatile styrene monomers have been detected from shell eggs stored for two weeks in polystyrene containers. Eggs contaminated in this manner may contain seven times more ethylbenzene and styrene, compared to fresh farm eggs not packaged this way.
- The benzene from multilayer, oxygen-barrier laminated bags can migrate into food—including meat, poultry and cheeses.
- While polyethylene used for food freezer bags and wraps does not contain plasticizers, printing applied to its surface can yield contaminating compounds during microwaving.
- Serious contamination might occur when plastic containers for carry-out foods are re-used and microwaved.
- Polyethylene terephthalate (PET), a popular plastic film wrap, allows the migration of adhesive components into foods during cooking with oils or foods that come in contact with the film.

Such radical transformation of the contemporary diet has been accelerated by self-serving corporate interests. Senator Gaylord Nelson (1972) issued this warning about the "food-industrial complex" three decades ago:

"The chemical and drug industries have joined the food industry in a food-industrial complex that the FDA is supposed to regulate. The result is a proliferation of food chemicals that are unnecessary, and unknown numbers that are unsafe, many of them untested, and most of them poorly monitored, at best."

Cultural Factors

There also has been greater recognition of cultural factors involving the diet that have potential neurotoxic consequences. The amyotrophic lateral sclerosis-parkinsonism-dementia syndrome among the Chamorros people on Guam, who consume a plant neurotoxin present in the *Cycad* species, provides a classic illustration (Spencer 1987). (This dwindling Guamanian disease has been referred to as "the Rosetta Stone of neurodegenerative disease.") Similar insights may help clarify the issue of "familial" AD (Chapter 3)—that is, its relationship to group dietary habits, especially early in life, rather than an autonomous genetic inheritance.

EXCESSIVE SUGAR CONSUMPTION

The intake of table sugar (sucrose) and other sugars used in "foods of commerce" rose dramatically during the second half of the 20th Century (Yudkin 1963, Antar 1964, Hodges 1965). At the same time, consumption of complex carbohydrates (chiefly as cereals and vegetables) was lower. Many persons currently consume annually the equivalent of their body weight in sugar!

The progressive increase per capita of total caloric intake from cane, beet and corn sweeteners, as well as low-calorie and non-caloric sweeteners, is reported from time to time by the Economic Research Service of the U.S. Department of Agriculture in *Sugar and Sweetener Reports*. The data are summarized in Table 7-1. It is paradoxical that the increased use of non-caloric and low-calorie sweeteners has not stopped the escalation of sugar consumption (Roberts 1989a).

PER CAPITA CONSUMPTION OF CALORIC AND LOW CALORIC SWEETENERS IN THE UNITED STATES

Year	Total Caloric (pounds)	Total Aspartame (pounds)	Total Saccharin (pounds)	Total of All (pounds)
1970	122.6	0	5.8	128.4
1975	118.1	0	6.1	124.2
1980	125.1	0	7.7	132.8
1985	130.9	12.0	6.0	142.4
1990	134.6	14.0	6.0	152.4

Table 7-1

Potentially neurotoxic chemicals are added to many sweet products as preservatives, flavorings and emulsifiers. Ice cream illustrates this issue. (The average American consumed 16 quarts in 1967.) It no longer consists only of milk, eggs and sugar. Referring to ice cream as "a chemical nightmare," Jerry Hoover (1993) listed the following synthetic chemicals that have been detected by analysis in "this dessert of kings":

- diethyl glycol as an emulsifier in place of eggs (also found in anti-freeze and paint removers)
- peperonal for replacing vanilla (also used to kill lice)
- aldehyde C17 for flavoring cherry ice cream (also found in aniline dyes, plastic and rubber)
- ethyl acetate for providing a pineapple flavor (also used as a cleaner for leather and textiles)
- butyraldehyde for nut flavoring (also used in rubber cement)
- amyl acetate for banana flavoring (also used as an oil paint solvent)
- benzyl acetate for strawberry flavoring (also a nitrate solvent)

The progressive increase in consumption of sugar and highly processed grains during the 20th Century has contributed to the frequency and severity of hyperinsulinemia and reactive hypoglycemia (Roberts 1964, 1968b, 1971b). Affected individuals are uniquely vulnerable to the ensuing clinical ravages caused by depletion of energy within the brain (Chapter 8).

The high consumption of sugary "junk foods" by children (Morgan 1981) is especially noteworthy. Of all age groups, children are the largest consumers of sugar. This matter is of particular concern relative to the potential severity of metabolic and neurologic complications. Some "children's cereals"—perhaps more accurately called "breakfast candies"—contain as many as 12 grams (3 teaspoons) of sugar per ounce.

The refining of raw sugar also results in a loss of important nutrients needed for its proper metabolism. They include chromium, manganese, cobalt, copper, zinc and magnesium (Hunter 1977). Deficits of these minerals have been reported to incur significant adverse medical and neurological consequences.

EXCESSIVE FRUCTOSE CONSUMPTION

Consumption of high-fructose corn syrup (HFCS) increased nearly <u>tenfold</u> between 1975 and 1985 (Best 1987). The targeted marketing of fructose for obese persons and diabetic patients accelerated this trend, as did the partial or total replacement of table sugar (sucrose) by corn sweeteners in processed foods—e.g., soft drinks, confectionery products, frozen desserts, bakery products, and other processed foods.

High fructose intake tends to trigger excessive secretion of insulin... with the potential for severe cerebral glucopenia (Chapter 8). Such diets can adversely affect nervous system function through altered copper and iron metabolism (Holbrook 1989).

> A significant increase in absorption of iron occurs when healthy subjects ingest fructose, presumably due to its chelation within the alkaline medium of the duodenum (Brodan 1967). (It does not occur with glucose or sucrose). The potential neurotoxicity of iron is reviewed in Chapter 9.

Several groups of investigators also have demonstrated that fructose consumption by hyperinsulinemic persons—in the range of 15 percent of energy intake—results in significantly elevated total cholesterol and low-density-lipoprotein (LDL) cholesterol (Swanson 1992, Hallfrisch 1993).

EXCESSIVE CONSUMPTION OF HIGHLY PROCESSED GRAINS

The increased use of finely milled flour is pertinent. Particle size of wheat and corn influences the rate of their digestion and metabolism—i.e., reduced size leads to faster digestion.

A greater insulin response is elicited from eating finely ground wheat flour and fine cornmeal products, compared to those from whole grains, coarse wheat flour, and whole or cracked cornmeal (Heaton 1988).

EXCESSIVE CONSUMPTION OF PROTEIN

The intake of excessive protein and amino acids can adversely affect brain function by several mechanisms:

- Competition with important neurotransmitters (Chapters 5 and 9)
- Decreased availability of the uncommon D-form mirror images (stereoisomers) of amino acids (see below)
- Neurotoxic amino acid byproducts that result from overheating food (see below)
- Excessive intake of iron (Chapter 9)
- Excessive secretion of insulin (Chapter 8)

The current annual consumption of animal protein foods in the United States consists of 65 pounds of beef and veal, 63 pounds of poultry, and 49 pounds of pork. The total average of 178 pounds of these animal foods is higher than the estimated 137 pounds in 1955 (Durning 1991).

The use of considerable animal protein is also closely linked with excess fat intake. A shift to protein obtained from vegetables, nuts and legumes is therefore desirable (Chapter 18).

INCREASED INTAKE OF AMINO ACIDS AND THEIR STEREOISOMERS

Amino acids are frequently described as "the building blocks of protein." The common ones number 22; of these, 12 are termed "essential" for a proper diet—i.e., they must be obtained from food.

Amino acid intake increased during the 20th Century through the consumption of more meat, other protein foods, and amino acid products. For example, aspartame (NutraSweet®) (Chapter 9) is comprised of 50 percent phenylalanine and 40 percent aspartic acid, two amino acids.

Numerous observations concerning amino acids and related substances are germane. These are a few:

- Blood amino acid levels tend to increase with age, especially among women (Caballero 1991).
- There is a high affinity of human brain capillaries for phenylalanine (Choi 1986, Pardridge 1987).
- Several amino acids—especially aspartate, glutamate, and *N*-acetylaspartylglutamate—are involved in both learning and remembering (Spiers 1987).
- Aspartate binding of nerve cell membranes is decreased in the brain of AD patients (Procter 1986).

The Issue of Stereoisomers

Technologic developments have led to an increased consumption of uncommon stereoisomers or "mirror images" of important amino acids. These dextro (or D-form) amino acids—e.g., D-phenylalanine; D-aspartic acid; D-proline—are converted from the natural levo (or L-form) amino acids.

D-form amino acids are significant here because of their lessened or altered metabolism by the brain and other organs. This is reflected as lessened bioavailability, decreased digestibility, and interference with metabolic activities involving the more common L-form amino acids. For example, the D-isomers of amino acids exit slower from the brain than the L-isomers (Lajtha 1962), and presumably accumulate. I previously reviewed this subject (Roberts 1989a, 1992b).

Milk, meat, grain proteins and other foods undergo similar alterations in processing. The various processes include pasteurization, ultrapasteurization, homogenization, condensation, "velvetization," and microwaving (see below). Whereas condensed or evaporated milk produced by heating contains three percent D-aspartic acid, D-aspartic acid rises to 31 percent after the milk is heated to 230 C for 20 minutes—more than a tenfold increase!

The neurotoxicity of D-phenylalanine and D-aspartic acid at high levels will be discussed in Chapter 9. Here, I wish to note *the correlation of D-aspartic acid with aging in warm-blooded animals* (Man 1983), and to emphasize *the considerable relevance of this phenomenon to Alzheimer's disease.*

> A clinical clue is the severe confusion and memory loss experienced by persons who consume products containing aspartame (NutraSweet®) (Chapter 9). This synthesized chemical compound contains 40 percent aspartic acid. The amino acid undergoes conversion (racemization) during heating or prolonged storage.

EXCESSIVE HEATING OF FOODS

The nutritional problems and other health risks that can result from excessively heated foods are relevant. These methods include (1) dark roasting, smoking, charring and burning, (2) the use of charcoal, wood or gas as fuels in grilling and barbecuing foods, and (3) the non-enzymatic browning and caramelization of food (the Maillard reaction) (Hunter 1984). Also, microwaving of food has radically transformed contemporary eating habits and nutrition. When microwave and baking are modest, there tends to be minimal loss of vitamins, minerals and vegetable fat content.

Other factory technologies differ from conventional cooking methods—e.g., extrusion cooking, explosion puffing, and "instantization." These techniques utilize extreme temperatures and pressures, or repeated wetting and drying. A wide range of convenient long-shelf-life foods and novel snack products that require minimal home preparation are made possible by such processings. However, they are fraught with potential hazards, such as poor bioavailability, and the risks of neurotoxicity and cancer.

- The browning of protein foods decreases protein digestibility, chiefly due to the cross linkages formed between amino acid residues. Several amino acids (including lysine, tryptophan and glutamic acid) are rendered less available.

- The heterocyclic aromatic amines that result from reactions of the amino acids and creatinine (present in animal foods) have raised the specter of carcinogenicity.

Only a few examples of the profound changes effected by heating basic foods will be reviewed here.

Heating of Milk and Milk Products

Conventional pasteurization at 161°F and "ultrapasteurization" (also called flash pasteurization) induce changes in milk and cream. Ultrapasteurization at 280°F extends the shelf life of milk and cream, but denatures the protein... a tradeoff not recognized by consumers.

The L-phenylalanine in milk is transformed to its D-stereoisomer (see above) by heat treatment. A similar change occurs when infant formulas are microwaved. Such alterations might interfere with neurotransmitter function (Chapter 5).

The widespread use of milk pasteurized at ultrahigh temperatures is evident in Europe where the poor quality of many home refrigerators encouraged development of this line of milk that could be stored six months or longer without spoiling. Parmalat Finanziaria S.p.A. of Milan, the world's largest maker of UHT milk, projected sales of $2 billion during 1993 (*The New York Times* June 26, 1993, p. 19).

Heating Carbohydrates

Grains and potatoes (white and sweet) must be cooked. The ingestion of cooked native starches, however, tends to exaggerate the release of insulin and lessen the body's ability to metabolize glucose ("body sugar") (Chapter 8). Bornet et al (1989) reported these changed responses in healthy subjects who ingested such starches (e.g., wheat and peas) either raw, as starch gels (boiled and cooked), or when cooked and cooled after preliminary industrial processing.

Heating Orange Juice

The pasteurization of orange juice suffers similar alteration. Freshly squeezed orange juice contains considerable <u>active</u> ascorbic acid (*Consumer Reports* August 1976). But pasteurization degrades much of the L-ascorbic acid, its main anti-scorbutic active form, to dehydro-L-ascorbic acid.

DECLINE OF BREAST-FEEDING

The decline of breast-feeding, chiefly through emphasis on the virtues and convenience of infant formulas based on cow's milk, represents another profound nutritional change during this century.

The importance of breast-feeding for optimal development of the infant brain is widely acknowledged. For example, the associated stimulation of thyroid hormones during the first few weeks of life can be critical.

Scientists continue to find important bioactive compounds in breast milk that do not exist, or are present only minimally, in infant formulas. They include DHA (an omega-3 fatty acid that is highly concentrated in the brain and retina), mucin (a protein that suppresses the reproduction of rotavirus, a major cause of infant diarrhea), epidermal growth factor, prostaglandins and prolactin (Brody 1994).

The problem is compounded when infant formulas are heated excessively. For example, formulas microwaved for 10 minutes contain <u>cis</u>-isomers of hydroxyproline in concentrations of 1-2 mg/L, and D-proline which is known to be neurotoxic (Lubec 1989). This kind of alteration in protein and peptides might initiate or aggravate structural, functional and immunologic abnormalities.

SYNTHETIC FOODS AND FOOD ADDITIVES

Many potentially neurotoxic novel foods and food additives have not been adequately tested before marketing, especially when submitted by processors in the Generally Recognized As Safe (GRAS) category. Even if tested in animals, they infrequently were extensively tested in humans for prolonged periods.

The widespread consumption of aspartame and monosodium glutamate (Chapter 9) emphasizes this serious regulatory deficiency by federal agencies. Furthermore, the dramatic rise in additives for a wide range of products, particularly soft drinks, is projected to accelerate (Thayer 1991).

Additionally, our society is inundated with substitute or synthetic foods and fruit drinks, largely because processors realize substantial savings. These products include replacer cheese and tomato sauce; imitation chocolate-flavored foods and beverages; non-dairy creamers that contain no cream; imitation cherries; and synthetic orange drinks (Hunter 1977). The latter not only contain considerable table sugar (sucrose), but also synthetic colorings and flavorings of doubtful safety.

PRIOR MALNUTRITION AND STARVATION

Malnutrition in infancy and childhood represents a risk factor for the subsequent development of AD and other degenerative neurologic disorders. Both clinical experience and a vast literature on early malnutrition indicate the serious injury that malnutrition can inflict on the developing central nervous system, especially during the first two years.

These observations illustrate the problem:

- Early malnutrition has been found to adversely affect the learning ability and behavior of experimental animals (Barnes 1968).

- Infants under six months of age recovering from severe protein deficiency (kwashiorkor) have been found not to recoup their mental age deficit during the recovery period (Cravioto 1965). When the severe nutritional insult occurred at one to four years of age, the complications included reduced responsiveness to stimulation, inability to perform, and impaired learning.

Winick (1969) emphasized the *permanent* brain injury suffered by malnourished infants. He underscored the potential for a vicious cycle affecting subsequent generations in these terms:

"Research evidence suggests that undernutrition, especially during early infancy, may retard the growth and development of the brain. This produces a permanent effect that sets in motion a vicious cycle … It is among growing children then—especially in the young infant—that malnutrition is most dangerous."*

Concern about prior malnutrition also applies to adults. Henderson (1990) summarized studies linking AD with previous severe malnutrition or frank starvation. The subjects included former inmates of concentration and prisoner-of-war camps

PURPOSEFUL CALORIC DEPRIVATION

Severe caloric restriction and other forms of nutritional deprivation is widespread, especially among young adults. Many weight-conscious girls and women literally deny themselves food due to "fear of fat" (Roberts 1989a, 1992b).

- Our society is bombarded by sophisticated ads for diet sodas that unequivocally emphasize a preference for slimness. The element of deception, however, is illustrated by displaying models endowed with genetically-determined physiques that exist in less than five percent of the general population.

- "The Pepsi Generation" of young adults increasingly consumes more low-calorie cola beverages than coffee in the morning.

Many persons do not realize the vital importance of adequate fat. This is particularly true for women, who need 12 percent to survive famine, compared to three precent for men. Similarly, increased body fat is necessary for normal fertility and gestation—that is, at least 20 percent body fat.

A profound reduction of calories tends to increase the release of endorphins and enkephalins (peptides in the body with opiate-like activity). These natural substances also regulate glucose, as evidenced by a significant rise of plasma insulin and glucose concentrations (Giugliano 1987). The latter can contribute to clinical hypoglycemia and insulin resistance (Chapter 8).

*©1969 *Roche Medical Image & Commentary*. Reproduced with permission.

8

THE ROLE OF "HYPOGLYCEMIA"

Dainty dishes... create distempers of soul and body.

Philo
(Special Laws)

Because glucose is the major energy source for the brain, and none of this carbohydrate can be stored in the central nervous system, acute or chronic disruption of glucose metabolism (characteristic of diabetes) could be expected to influence cognitive functioning.*

Clarissa S. Holmes (1987)

The brain requires an adequate and continuous supply of glucose ("body sugar") for proper functioning. This fact *must* be considered in any degenerative brain disease.

Persons who have witnessed a severe insulin reaction, or who have experienced an attack of reactive hypoglycemia ("low blood sugar"), can affirm that serious cerebral dysfunction occurs when the brain is deprived of sufficient glucose. I have elaborated upon this issue and its clinical significance in many publications (Roberts 1964, 1965, 1966, 1967, 1966a, 1969, 1973b).

It is my belief, based on considerable observation and research, that severe recurrent depletion of brain glucose (cerebral glucopenia) constitutes a major factor in the evolution of Alzheimer's disease (AD). Only a portion of the evidence can be reviewed here.

> Historically, prominent physiologists and neurologists suspected the central role of energy depletion within the brain as the cause of some degenerative brain diseases. In 1908, one year after the report by Alzheimer, Elie Metchnikoff wrote in *The Prolongation of Life*: "In senile degeneration, the cells are surrounded by neuronophages which absorb their contents and bring about more or less complete atrophy."

**©1987 American Diabetes Association. Reproduced from *Diabetes Care* with permission.

Recent investigators have expressed similar views, albeit in more technical terms. Bowmen et al (1979) concluded that AD primarily represents a degenerative nerve cell disorder characterized by "a selective reduction in all glycolytic enzymes involved in hexosemonophosphate metabolism."

BRAIN GLUCOSE REQUIREMENTS, METABOLISM
AND HOMEOSTASIS

The brain of an average-sized individual requires about 112 grams (gm) glucose daily. For comparison, red blood cells, which also are dependent on glucose, require only 35 gm daily.

Defenses Against Hypoglycemia (Cerebral Glucopenia)

Nature has endowed humans with extraordinary mechanisms to ensure adequate energy for the brain from glucose.

- Glucose moves freely across the membranes of nerve cells to sustain their metabolism. Indeed, brain capillary cells transport ten times their weight of glucose per minute to meet cerebral glucose requirements.

- The transfer of glucose from blood into the brain is facilitated by a unique diffusion system. It entails the combination of glucose with a membrane carrier or transporter. The demonstration by Kalaria and Harik (1989) of reduced glucose-transporter protein within the brain microvessels, hippocampus and neocortex of AD patients is especially significant in view of the decreased glucose uptake in these regions noted by positron emission tomography (PET) and other imaging studies (Chapter 4). Furthermore, such glucose transporter reduction is *unrelated* to age.

- Nerve cells possess a remarkable mechanism, known as the Krebs cycle, which enables them to oxidize glucose completely to carbon dioxide and water.

- Sensitive glucose receptors exist within the brain that warn it of impending glucose depletion.

- Multiple counterregulatory mechanisms, involving hormonal responses and neurogenic reflexes, also serve as protective defenses against impending cerebral glucopenia. These mechanisms include the release of cortisone, glucagon, growth hormone, epinephrine and norepinephrine, and stimulation of the autonomic (automatic) nervous system.

Unfortunately, many of the foregoing mechanisms are limited and transient.

- The protection against hypoglycemia by hormonal responses has limitations, even among normal persons. This may not be appreciated from studies involving single episodes of induced hypoglycemia. Davis and Shamoon (1991) reported decreased glucose output from the liver in response to a second hypoglycemic event during identical degrees of hypoglycemia. There was also a reduction in plasma glucagon, growth hormone and cortisone responses.

- There is reduced release of counterregulatory hormones (epinephrine; growth hormone; glucagon) among insulin-dependent diabetics in response to severe hypoglycemia (Diamond 1991). This poses a great danger when such patients receive large doses of insulin for "tight control," but fail to take adequate interval feedings, especially at night.

- Glucose does not penetrate the brain as rapidly at diminished circulating glucose concentrations than at normal levels (Butterfield 1966).

- Hypoglycemia markedly reduces the ability of blood vessels in the brain to dilate (Gomez 1992). Therefore, a reduction in cerebral blood flow can compound the glucopenic insult.

- Recent hypoglycemia can result in decreased recognition of hypoglycemia by the brain, and the decreased secretion of major counterregulatory hormones, notably glucagon and epinephrine (Hoeldtke 1994). Accordingly, the individual may fail to perceive subsequent hypoglycemic attacks.

MECHANISMS AND EFFECTS OF CEREBRAL GLUCOPENIA

Severe reduction of glucose to the brain (cerebral glucopenia) can cause marked alterations in neurons, their supporting (glial) cells, and the nerve sheath (myelin).

One major mechanism by which hypoglycemia causes or contributes to brain damage is the induction of *glutamate and aspartate neurotoxicity* (Chapter 9). These excitatory amino acids stimulate the N-methyl-D-aspartate (NMDA) receptor. In turn, NMDA increases intracellular calcium… believed to be an important mechanism for causing selective nerve cell death in AD.

- Mattson et al (1993) reviewed the important role of the calcium ion (Ca^{++}) in regulating nerve structure and function. It is also a convergence point for multiple initiating causes of nerve injury involving disturbed amyloid metabolism (Chapter 4) and the overactivity of glutamatergic systems.

- Calcium mediates adaptive changes in the cytoarchitecture of neurons—including neurite outgrowth, synaptic remodeling, and natural cell death—in response to environmental signals such as occur in trauma, stroke and AD.

- Calcium influx can result from glutamate's effect as an excitotoxin, especially under the conditions of hypoglycemia and hypoxia.

- During and Spencer (1993) documented a rise in extracellular glutamate prior to spontaneous seizures in the conscious human brain.

The role of hypoglycemia and tissue glucopenia in increasing oxidative stress is indicated by the demonstration that glucose and other simple sugars have peroxy radical quenching properties (Wehmeier 1993). (This property is shared with ascorbate, a potent water-soluble antioxidant.) The mechanisms may be both direct and indirect, such as through an action on glycosylation reaction.

Areas Uniquely Vulnerable to Glucopenia

Certain areas within the nervous system are highly susceptible to glucose deprivation. It is manifest by the AD brain as <u>bilateral and symmetric deficits in glucose metabolism involving the temporal lobes</u> (see below).

The <u>hippocampus</u> (Chapter 4), which plays a crucial role in memory and mental clarity, is another vulnerable site. The metabolic uniqueness of the hippocampal formation involving altered cytochrome oxidase activity has been demonstrated by Simonian and Hyman (1993).

- Cytochrome oxidase is the terminal enzyme of the electron transport chain by which tissues obtain energy. Its activity in neurons correlates with nerve impulse input, tending to be diminished with decreased afferent activity.

- These investigators could not detect the distinct dark band of cytochrome oxidase activity that is normally found in the outer two-thirds of the molecular layer of the dentate gyrus, final zone of the so-called perforant pathway.

<u>Specific nerve tracts</u> also are sensitive to glucopenia. For example, an important enzyme, glucose-6-phosphate dehydrogenase, is four times more concentrated in heavily myelinated central tracts than in lightly myelinated ones (McDougal 1961, 1964). This explains, in part, the localization of changes within corticospinal tracts of the spinal cord in multiple sclerosis (Roberts 1966b,c).

Prematurity and Low Birth Weight

These factors increase the ravages of hypoglycemia on the brain. Haworth and McRae (1965) commented: "… it is hardly surprising that lack of glucose substrate for vital oxidative processes, and for the synthesis of raw materials for incorporation into new nervous tissue, should result in neurological symptoms."

"FUNCTIONAL" (DIABETOGENIC) HYPERINSULINISM

An associated major risk factor for AD is repeated cerebral glucopenia over prolonged periods resulting from the secretion of excessive insulin. At least one-third of the general population has this genetically-influenced disorder. It has been variously termed "functional" hyperinsulinism and "diabetogenic" hyperinsulinism (Roberts 1964, 1965, 1966, 1967, 1968a).

- The term "functional" indicates that the hypoglycemia is <u>not</u> caused by a pancreatic tumor that produces insulin. (In practice, such tumors are *rare.*)

- The term "diabetogenic" signifies a continuum involving the effects of recurring and excessive strain upon the insulin-producing islet cells of the pancreas. The ensuing depletion of insulin reserve can progress to the point of being unable to handle a sugar load—referred to as <u>decreased glucose tolerance.</u> This results in the progressive wasting and lessened efficacy of insulin ("insulin resistance")… and ultimately, overt diabetes mellitus.

Individuals with this trait release considerable insulin in response to sugars (sucrose;

glucose; fructose; galactose), protein, amino acids, large meals, and other influences.

A "hypoglycemic attack" tends to occur several hours after eating. Typically, it is characterized by profound weakness (e.g., "draining of my strength," "sapping of my energy," "late morning slump," "afternoon letdown"), intense hunger, "nervousness," headache, sweats, severe shaking (tremor), and a craving for food—especially sugar. The reaction generally subsides after eating or taking sugar. The true nature of such attacks, particularly during the night, might not be recognized for prolonged periods.

Diabetogenic hyperinsulinism (DH) is widespread. This phenomenon is largely explainable by the survival nature of its "thrifty gene" (Neel 1965), especially during periods of starvation. In particular, this genetic influence enabled primitive man to deposit more fat reserves whenever food became scarce. There is a caveat in converse: the serious neurologic and other complications of severe caloric restriction, especially by weight-conscious girls and women (Chapters 7 and 18).

Neurologic, Cognitive and Psychiatric Features

The numerous neurologic and psychiatric manifestations of hypoglycemia reflect severe metabolic stress upon brain function. The symptoms include dizziness (vertigo), unsteady gait, double vision, tingling or related nerve sensations (paresthesias), and inability to think clearly or to verbalize properly. If unchecked, severe hypoglycemia might induce epileptiform seizures, unconsciousness, psychopathic behavior, or a psychotic state.

An immediate hazard of inadequate glucose supply to the brain is loss of cognitive function (Amiel 1993). Even small decreases in the blood glucose concentration elicit counterregulatory protective responses. They include decreased secretion of endogenous insulin, activation of the sympathetic nervous system, and release of glucose-elevating hormones (glucagon, cortisol, catecholamines). The problem becomes accentuated with a defective counterregulatory response that results in "unawareness of hypoglycemia." Furthermore, a vicious cycle occurs because hypoglycemia itself can induce such counterregulatory defects. The problem of unrecognized hypoglycemia is significant among diabetic patients who receive intensive insulin therapy (Amiel 1993).

Many investigators have confirmed the association between hypoglycemia and altered cognition, often without affecting gross motor performance. These are a few:

- Jones et al (1990) evaluated the effect of mild hypoglycemia on brain function in healthy adults by measuring responses known as brain stem and auditory evoked potentials. Even modest reductions in circulating glucose were associated with markedly altered responses to auditory stimuli.

- Haier (1988) correlated psychological function with glucose metabolism in the brain by positron emission tomography (PET).

- Blackman et al (1990) reported abnormal decision-making by healthy adult volunteers during insulin-induced hypoglycemia.

- Holmes (1987) noted transient impairment of cognition—viz., alterations of decision-making, speed to recall, and verbal fluency—in adult diabetics tested during and after clinical hypoglycemia.

Several investigators have documented higher insulin levels in both the blood and cerebrospinal fluid in AD patients after drinking glucose (Bucht 1983, Fujisawa 1991).

Glucose Tolerance Testing

The clinical diagnosis of reactive hypoglycemia due to functional hyperinsulinism, with or without associated "chemical diabetes," generally can be confirmed by properly performed oral glucose tolerance testing. This procedure entails drinking a sufficient amount of glucose, and measuring glucose levels for four to six hours, with or without concomitant measurement of circulating insulin concentrations. I have previously elaborated upon the details and diagnostic criteria of both morning and afternoon testing (Roberts 1964a, 1968a, 1971b).

The responses of such a patient are shown in Figure 8-1. Noteworthy are the intensification of reactive hypoglycemia and the decrease of glucose tolerance later in the day.

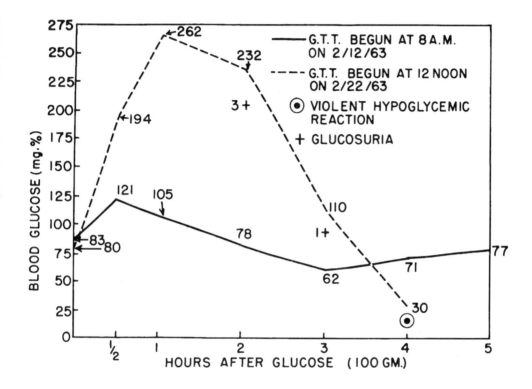

Figure 8-1

Comparative responses during morning and afternoon glucose tolerance testing in a 38-year-old female with symptomatic reactive hypoglycemia and a paternal history of diabetes mellitus. Note the intensification of reactive hypoglycemia during the afternoon, and the documentation of decreased glucose tolerance *only* by the afternoon study.

I described the cyclic acceleration of insulin release during the afternoon and evening in previous publications (Roberts 1964a, 1968b). Others (Lambert 1966; Bowen 1967; Jarrett 1969) have verified this phenomenon.

The tendency for hypoglycemia to be more severe during the evening or early morning hours offers clinical insights applicable to the behavior of both AD-prone persons and AD patients. This could explain in part their increased confusion at night, early morning awakenings, night wandering, nocturnal visual or auditory hallucinations, rapid movements of the limbs or body (myoclonic jerks), and so-called "sundowning" (altered behavior and cognition as evening approaches).

The Issue of "Hypoglycemia Bias"

Notwithstanding its considerable clinical importance and public health implications, much bias exists among many physicians who are reluctant to make a diagnosis of "reactive hypoglycemia." These are a few of the reasons:

- Denigration of this disorder stemming from dogmas expressed by teachers and "authorities"

- Failure even to consider and pursue the diagnosis of hypoglycemia in clinically appropriate settings

- Failure to understand the severe limitations of current diagnostic methods, especially conventional morning glucose tolerance testing (see above)

The symptoms of "hypoglycemia" reflect the direct and indirect effects of decreased glucose concentrations *in the brain and other tissues* rather than the blood. Accordingly, circulating glucose concentrations at such times might not be diagnostically low. This is consistent with (1) the findings of my correlative biochemical-electroencephalographic studies in patients with diabetogenic hyperinsulinism (Roberts 1964a,b, 1971b), and (2) the counterregulatory responses (see above) that serve to elevate glucose levels. Adamkiewicz (1963) observed: "It is assumed that the degree of blood glycemia is a reflection of a degree of glycemia in all the body fluids. This assumption has important limitations. For example, blood glycemia may not necessarily reflect the rapid local changes of glycemia in the interstitial fluids that bathe the cell walls."

OTHER PERTINENT ASPECTS OF "FUNCTIONAL" HYPERINSULINISM

The following aspects of functional hyperinsulinism are noteworthy because they help explain certain aspects of Alzheimer's disease noted by others.

Relationship to Gender

Females seem disproportionately afflicted with AD (Chapters 2 and 16), even when their greater longevity and other possible explanations have been considered. Elderly women also are more prone to diabetogenic hyperinsulinism (Zeytinoglu 1969).

These are some of the probable underlying hormonal influences operative in females.

- Diethylstilbestrol (a female hormone drug) depresses glucose oxidation in brain tissue (Gordon 1947).

- Women experience more severe reactive hypoglycemia under certain hormonally-related circumstances—including the premenstrual period, the first half of pregnancy, and while using birth-control drugs ("the pill").

Relationship to Aging

Diabetogenic hyperinsulinism tends to become exaggerated with aging. This has been documented during oral glucose tolerance testing in the elderly (Metz 1966, Shima 1967, Zeytinoglu 1969).

Furthermore, the aging process is associated with diminished ability to recover from hypoglycemia due to lessened counterregulatory hormonal responses (see above), especially glucagon and epinephrine release (Ortiz 1992). The hyperinsulinemia and decreased glucose tolerance associated with aging also could be related to changes in regional body fat distribution (Coon 1992).

With reference to confusion and memory loss, the association between aging and DH or non-insulin-dependent diabetes is germane. Older patients with these disorders tend to have greater deficits in processing complex verbal and nonverbal material even when they appear to be functioning well (Reaven 1990).

Relationship to Race

I reported the higher frequency and greater severity of diabetogenic hyperinsulinism among African Americans, especially women (Roberts 1964a). Others have confirmed this phenomenon. Data showing an increased prevalence of AD among hospitalized blacks (May 1991), and in several regional surveys —e.g., Mississippi (Schoenberg 1985)—underscore the relevance of this subject.

Relationship to Smoking

Tobacco hypoglycemia is a recognized entity (Roberts 1971b). Persons who habitually smoke one pack or more of cigarettes daily tend to release excessive insulin in response to glucose (Szanto 1968). Insulin release declined significantly when such persons were tested after they stopped smoking for two weeks.

Relationship to Weight Gain

Many investigators have affirmed that progressive hyperinsulinemia is associated with weight gain. This is especially significant among middle-aged women (Wing 1992).

Relationship to Family History

There are striking familial ramifications of DH and its complications. Wing et al (1992) emphasized the significance of a parental history of either diabetes or hypertension relative to elevated plasma insulin levels, which is independent of the body mass index. The highest insulin concentrations were noted when parents had both diseases.

Relationship to Other Clinical Risk Factors Associated With AD (Section III)

The clinical ramifications of hypoglycemia have considerable relevance to many of the phenomena encountered in the AD-prone state. They include migraine (Roberts 1967d), angina pectoris (Roberts 1966g, 1967a, 1991b), palpitations (Roberts 1967a, 1971b), leg cramps (Roberts 1965a, 1973), and seizures (Roberts 1964a,b, 1971b).

DECREASED CEREBRAL GLUCOSE UPTAKE IN ALZHEIMER'S DISEASE

Energy-related metabolism within the AD-prone brain is considerably altered prior to the onset of dementia, and probably before the development of many neurofibrillary tangles and senile plaques (Chapter 4). A variety of methods, both invasive and noninvasive, have demonstrated the decrease of glucose oxidation in the AD brain, especially within the parietal and frontal areas where the pathophysiology is most prominent. Furthermore, there tends to be a quantitative correlation of such metabolic defects with the degree of dementia.

- Khachaturian (1989) suspected that the neurochemical deficits found in AD result from disturbances in nerve cells "such as abnormal oxidative or glucose metabolism."

- Friedland et al (1988b) reported that "… metabolic abnormalities can precede nonmemory neuropsychologic deficits by years, and predict the pattern of neuropsychologic deficits eventually seen."

- Hoyer (1993) reported reductions of brain glucose utilization and ATP formation of 54% and 81%, respectively, in AD brains, compared to control values. Such reductions reduce the availability of the glucose-derived neurotransmitter acetylcholine. Hoyer proposed that the diminished glucose utilization and energy shortage contribute significantly to abnormal amyloid precursor protein processing… and to subsequent amyloid formation.

Glucose metabolism is profoundly altered in specific regions of the AD brain. This has been demonstrated by imaging studies such as PET, which utilizes 2-[^{18}F] fluoro-2-deoxy-D-glucose as a positron source. Bilateral symmetric hypometabolism in the parietal-temporal association areas is noted in AD by this method (Mahler 1991) and by single photon emission tomography (SPECT). In contrast, multiple asymmetric regions of cortical and subcortical hypometabolism characterize multi-infarct dementia (MID) due to small strokes.

- Diminished metabolism in the temporal-parietal-occipital junction regions of both hemispheres has been found by PET *early* in the course of AD (Culter 1985).

- Hoyer (1991) studied cerebral glucose metabolism in patients with early-onset AD and late-onset AD. The predominant disturbance among patients with normal blood glucose concentrations in each category was a significant reduction of cerebral glucose utilization.

The causal role of reduced energy availability/utilization in AD is indicated by the

70

ability of hypoglycemia to elicit neurofibrillary tangle-like changes in hippocampal neurons (Cheng 1992, Mattson 1993). Reduced availability of glucose causes depletion of adenosine triphosphate (ATP), failure of the calcium ion extrusion/buffering systems, membrane depolarization, excess release of the excitotoxin glutamate, and activation of the NMDA receptor (see above).

These phenomenona are highly pertinent to vicious neuropathic cycles in crucial areas induced by recurrent severe hypoglycemia. Decreased glucose utilization by the AD brain ultimately reflects metabolic disturbances due to severe cerebral glucopenia and other causes, and the degeneration of nerve cells within severely affected areas. It may be compounded by several factors. They include reduced blood flow to the brain from occlusive vascular disease (Chapter 12), the presence of aluminum (Lipman 1989) (Chapter 10), and the effects of various neurotoxins (Chapters 9 and 11).

Mitochondrial Changes

There has been increased recognition that altered mitochondria significantly contribute to energy impairment in the AD brain. These granular or rod-shaped bodies play a critical role in cellular metabolism.

Blass (1993) reviewed the direct evidence of mitochondrial damage in the AD brain. It has been found not only in areas with demonstrable anatomic damage, but also in other areas that appear normal histologically. This is particularly true for the alpha-ketoglutarate dehydrogenase complex, which is reduced more than half compared to matched non-AD controls. (Such reduced activity limits the rate of glucose oxidation by the brain.)

Mitochondrial abnormalities also increase the vulnerability of brain cells to various stressors.

- Cultured neurons deprived of glucose are unable to survive the addition of a dose of glutamate that would have no significant effect when glucose was present (Henneberry 1989).

- Other investigators have demonstrated comparable cell death following glucose deprivation after the exposure of nerve cells to toxic fragments of APP, hypoxia, thiamine deficiency, or adrenal hormones.

- Mattson et al (1993) demonstrated the impaired ability of neuronal mitochondria to accumulate rhodamine-123 within 12-24 hours after the onset of hypoglycemia. ("Healthy" mitochondria accumulate this fluorescent dye, whereas impaired mitochondria do not.) Moreover, pretreatment of neurons with nerve growth factor (NGF) and basic fibroblast growth factor (bFGF) (Chapter 5) can prevent such mitochondrial dysfunction if given prior to the onset of hypoglycemia.

ROLE OF HYPOGLYCEMIA AND HYPERINSULINISM IN RELATED PHENOMENA

The depletion of glucose as a major energy source for tissues, coupled with the direct effects of excessive insulin, can contribute to other changes associated with development of AD. Much more research in these areas is required.

Depletion of "Cholinergic Reserve"

Glucose deprivation affects acetylcholine metabolism. Acetylcholine, a "cholinergic" compound released at nerve endings, is vital for the transmission of nerve impulses. Deficient cholinergic activity within the hippocampus and related structures of AD patients was discussed in Chapter 5.

Acetylcholine requires energy at various steps of its synthesis. Prolonged and recurrent hypoglycemia therefore could interfere with the functioning of this important neurotransmitter by damaging cholinergic neurons and depleting the "cholinergic reserve."

Increased Immune Responses

Some investigators believe that immune mechanisms, especially involving the supporting glial cells, play a significant role in AD (Chapter 6). Elsewhere, I have reviewed the intensification of immune responses by hypoglycemia (Roberts 1979a, 1993). Adamkiewicz (1963) stressed that hypoglycemia—whether resulting from fasting, insulin administration, or adrenalectomy—can potentiate anaphylactoid and allergic reactions.

Insulin and Amyloid

Diabetogenic hyperinsulinism may influence the deposition of amyloid (Chapter 4) in Alzheimer's disease. There also is amyloid deposition in diabetes mellitus. Although the amyloid in AD differs from that found in diabetes mellitus, some of the pathogenetic mechanisms may overlap.

> Amylin or islet amyloid polypeptide (IAPP) is a 37-amino-acid peptide. It can be detected within the extracellular amyloid in half the pancreatic islets of patients with non-insulin-dependent diabetes mellitus (NIDDM) (Butler 1990, Steiner 1991). This substance is secreted in response to ingested glucose or a mixed meal. It circulates at comparable concentrations in both nondiabetic subjects and NIDDM patients.

A correlation exists between amyloid A in insulin-dependent diabetes mellitus and excessive insulin levels (Brownlee 1984). Insulin delivered by a continuous subcutaneous pump increases serum amyloid A to levels nearly six times those found in control subjects, and nearly twice as much as when the insulin is given by intermittent subcutaneous injection.

Other observations support a likely overlap of the molecular defect(s) that predispose to amyloid deposition in both pancreatic islet cells and brain. Laedtke et al (1994) reported a significantly higher incidence of glucose intolerance in a cohort of 100 AD patients compared to age-matched controls, notwithstanding a lower body mass index in the former.

9

THE ROLE OF DIETARY NEUROTOXINS

*Anecdotal reports of neurotoxicity in humans need to be pursued
vigorously with clinical surveillance and follow-up.*

The National Research Council (1991)
(Environmental Neurotoxicology)

*Finally, we should learn a lesson from the NutraSweet® experience.
If a food additive has potential neurological or behavioral
effects, it should undergo human clinical testing,
similar to the process a drug must undergo,
before it is put on the market.*

Senator Howard M. Metzenbaum (1987)

Chapter 7 provided an overview of the adverse effects of changes in the diet and eating habits that relate to the emergence of Alzheimer's disease (AD) as a contemporary epidemic. The neurotoxic effects of monosodium glutamate (MSG) and aspartame (NutraSweet®), two widely used additives, also warrant analysis because of related clinical problems and biochemical associations. The latter include amino acid changes within the amyloid plaques and neurofibrillary tangles that characterize this disease (Chapter 4). Similar considerations apply to phenylalanine and galactose consumption by the many "carriers" of several important inherited disorders.

For perspective, the United States has become more of an abusing rather than using nation. The wholesale ingestion of free amino acids during the latter half of the 20th Century is a case in point.

- Editorializing on the eosinophilia-myalgia syndrome precipitated by ingesting L-tryptophan, Duffy (1992) stressed that physicians should be better informed about the potential hazards of such consumer products… including the welfare of future generations.

- Dr. Irvin H. Rosenberg (1982) commented on the extraordinary marketing of products as foods or dietary supplements—not as drugs—in health-food stores and pharmacies with little or no clinical testing.

"Have the health-food stores become the foci of an alternative health system that claims to focus on health and the prevention of disease, while the medical profession is seen in caricature as being concerned only with drugs? One need only enter a health-food store and examine the shelves of products to learn that the health-food 'system,' too, depends heavily on pills and capsules; however, for regulatory purposes these are foods or dietary supplements. We must ask whether the response of physicians and scientific medical societies to the public's increasing appetite for nutritional information has been adequately informed and sufficiently concerned."*

The overstimulation of receptors for excitatory amino acids, including aspartate and glutamate, is believed to represent a "final common pathway" for both many acute neurologic disorders and chronic neurodegenerative states. Glutamate represents the principal excitatory neurotransmitter in the brain. Its interactions with specific membrane receptors affect cognition, memory, movement and sensation. Activation of glutamate receptors results in excessive influx of calcium into neurons, and subsequent neuronal injury. Lipton and Rosenberg (1994) reviewed the mechanisms.

MONOSODIUM GLUTAMATE (MSG)

Monosodium glutamate (MSG), the sodium salt of the amino acid glutamate (glutamic acid), has been widely incorporated in the food supply. Some of the flavorings and seasonings that contain this popular additive are Accent®, Zest®, Vestin®, Subu®, Glutavene®, and Lawry's Seasoning Salt®.

Up to 30 percent of persons in the United States are estimated to be adversely affected by taking manufactured glutamic acid in daily amounts of five grams or more (Kenney 1972, Reif-Lehrer 1976, Samuels 1991). Jack L. Samuels (1991) opined to the Federation of American Societies for Experimental Biology (FASEB) that at least 60 million persons in the United States may have reactions of varying severity to MSG. Some experience the typical "Chinese restaurant syndrome" after ingesting soup prepared with MSG. The ubiquity of MSG in food preparation, however, suggests "American restaurant syndrome" as a more appropriate term.

The neurotoxicity of glutamate contributes to brain damage in severe hypoglycemia (Chapter 8) and oxygen deprivation (Chapter 12).

General Considerations

Glutamate is an non-essential amino acid abundantly present in plant and animal protein. Reference to MSG sensitivity-toxicity in this discussion refers to <u>manufactured</u>

---

*©1982 *New England Journal of Medicine*. Reproduced with permission.

glutamic acid… not glutamic acid or glutamate found in unadulterated protein.

A sodium ion is added to manufacture MSG. After 1958, MSG was produced in large quantities by means of fermentating natural ingredients (corn; wheat; soybeans; sugar beets; sugar cane; tapioca starch; kelp; molasses).

One should appreciate the shortcomings of the term "flavor enhancer." MSG increases the perception of sweet and salty tastes by temporarily deadening the perception of bitterness. Unfortunately, this consumer-appealing influence removes an important biological defense mechanism aimed at detecting—and rejecting—spoiled or contaminated food.

Presence of MSG in Food and Other Products

The amount of MSG in an average serving of soup reconstituted from commercially available dry bases is 735 mg or 0.735 gm (*Consumer Reports* November 1978, pp. 615-169). Glutamate levels rise proportionate to the quantity of MSG consumed.

Many food products contain "hidden" monosodium glutamate. For example, it is a constituent of the hydrolyzed vegetable protein (HVP), also known as protein hydrolysate, present in numerous products. They include soups, luncheon meats, gravies, sauces, candy, chewing gum, soft drinks, binders for drugs, and "reaction flavors." (The reaction flavors are a mix of any protein material [e.g., milk, peanuts, seafood, gluten] and reduced sugar heated at high temperatures.)

Dr. Adrienne Samuels (1991) developed the following slightly-modified classification (reproduced with permission).

- These foods and additives always contain glutamate, including MSG:
    Monosodium glutamate
    Hydrolyzed protein
    Hydrolyzed oat flour
    Sodium caseinate
    Calcium caseinate
    Yeast extract
    Yeast nutrients
    Yeast food
    Autolyzed yeast
    Textured protein

- These foods and additives often contain MSG (amounts depending upon manufacturing conditions):
    Malt extract
    Malt flavoring
    Bouillon
    Barley salt
    Broth
    Stock
    Tomato paste
    Seasonings
    Flavoring(s)
    Natural flavoring(s)
    Natural beef flavoring

Natural chicken flavoring
Natural pork flavoring

- These enzymes create MSG:
Protease enzymes
Fungi protease
Protease

The FDA requires identification of glutamate as "monosodium glutamate" on food labels when hydrolyzed protein has been refined to approximately 99% glutamate. In lesser amounts, the product is termed "hydrolyzed protein products" (HPP). They include "calcium caseinate" (about 15%), "sodium caseinate" (about 15%), "autolyzed yeast and extract" (5-25%), and "hydrolyzed protein" and "hydrolyzed vegetable protein" (5-12%). There is presently no limit on the amount of MSG and related products that can be added to food.

The problem is compounded by (1) the denial of MSG sensitivity by corporate-funded "experts," and (2) the "name games" in labeling. The latter have forced MSG-sensitive persons to scrutinize and question every dish served in restaurants to avoid "trial by testing and illness." For example, "no MSG added" does NOT exclude its presence. Similarly, significant amounts can exist in "all natural" products. Finding flour that does not contain MSG has been a monumental challenge for some reactors.

Nature of Reactions

Clinical reactions to MSG usually involve multiple systems… the brain most dramatically. The neuropsychiatric symptoms include disorientation, confusion ("brain fatigue"), dizziness, depression, severe anxiety, headache, hyperactivity, sleepiness, insomnia, numbness, burning sensations, slurred speech, facial pressure and blurred vision. Other common complaints are severe flushing, a rash, extreme thirst, nausea, vomiting, abdominal cramps, diarrhea, chest pain, palpitations and asthmatic attacks.

As with reactors to aspartame products, other family members may suffer MSG reactions.

A number of MSG reactors also cannot tolerate aspartame products (see below). Some have commented on the similarity of their reactions to MSG and to aspartame. Moreover, the diagnosis of multiple sclerosis has been frequently made in patients with both types of sensitivity (Roberts 1989, 1993).

Neurotoxicity

Manufactured glutamic acid is a neurotoxin or so-called excitotoxin. (As a natural component of unadulterated foods, glutamic acid is bound to protein and well digested.) Its hydrolysis by the use of chemicals or enzymes releases L-glutamic acid, which can be neurotoxic in the free state. (MSG is effective as a flavor intensifier only in the free state.)

Couratier et al (1993) analyzed the modification of beta-amyloid (Chapter 4) produced by glutamate toxicity on primary neuronal cultures. They found that calcium-dependent glutamate toxicity induces a dose-dependent increase of beta-amyloid immunostaining, chiefly located on the plasma membrane and in neuronal debris.

The adverse effects of MSG in the young should be cause for considerable concern. Hydrolyzed protein products cause hypothalamic lesions and neuroendocrine dysfunction in neonatal primates (Olney 1973). When ingested by human infants, as previously occurred with commercial baby foods containing MSG and HVP, long-term adverse effects on brain function might develop. The administration of MSG to young rats decreases choline uptake by the frontal cortex of the brain, and reduces choline acyltransferase activity—effects resembling the changes associated with AD (Chapters 4 and 5).

> Dr. John Olney has repeatedly demonstrated such destruction of neurons in the immature hypothalamus within <u>minutes.</u> He further emphasized the erroneous assumption that gastrointestinal absorption of glutamate in man is the same as in animals because humans absorb much more (Olney 1993).

It is reasonable to infer that the prolonged consumption of neurotoxins, such as MSG and the amino acids in aspartame, might incur pathologic changes within the brain, the spinal cord, and elsewhere. Dr. Adrienne Samuels (1991) commented

> "Yet, in today's society, there is far more glutamate available to the average human being than has been given to any laboratory animal. There is the potential that, beginning as an infant, a human could consume considerable quantities of glutamate <u>daily.</u> Consumption could well continue through a lifetime, through periods of illness and stress (weakened immune system), and physical disability (torn muscle, tissue and bone) unknown to laboratory animals, and for periods of time far exceeding a single dose or ingestion over a period of 10 days or even three years. In no way do the animals studied directly parallel the human condition. The human potentially ingests more glutamate in one week than a laboratory animal would ever be exposed to." (Reproduced with permission)

The extensive critique of Dr. Samuels (1991) concluded that no study nor a preponderance of the literature "proves" the safety of manufactured free glutamate ingested in any form. Accordingly, disinformation about its safety issued by the FDA and corporate-funded scientists should be challenged in the face of a dramatic increase of Alzheimer's disease, Parkinson's disease, amyotropic lateral sclerosis (ALS), and other neurodegenerative conditions.

Pyridoxine deficiency appears to enhance the toxicity of MSG (*Nutrition Reviews* 1973; 31(2): 70-71).

ASPARTAME

Many persons have experienced severe confusion and memory loss after consuming products that contain aspartame (ASP), a low-calorie sweetener widely known as NutraSweet® and Equal®. These reactors offer a unique "experiment of Nature" that has extraordinary relevance to AD for two reasons. First, such reactions may constitute a reversible human model for studying "early" Alzheimer's disease. Second, this association provides fertile clues for preventing AD.

Aspartame is a synthesized compound. Its components include the two amino acids (referred to as "the building blocks of protein") <u>phenylalanine</u> (50%) and <u>aspartic acid</u> (40%), and a methyl ester. The chemical formula appears in Figure 9-1.

Both of these amino acids are problematic. Their significance is discussed below.

In the stomach, ASP promptly releases from the methyl ester about 10 percent <u>methyl alcohol</u> (methanol)... an unequivocal poison. This fact explains in part the eye reactions and some other symptoms experienced by persons who ingest large amounts of ASP products.

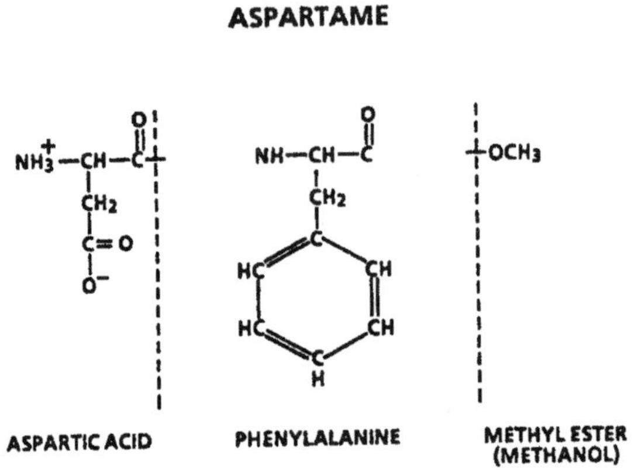

ASPARTAME

ASPARTIC ACID   PHENYLALANINE   METHYL ESTER (METHANOL)

Figure 9-1
The chemical formula of aspartame.

Also, striking chemical and physical changes of the ingredients occur whenever ASP products are heated or stored for long periods (Roberts 1989a, 1992b). They include the formation of several <u>stereoisomers</u> (mirror images) and <u>other potentially toxic breakdown products</u>; all are germane to the AD problem.

The enormous consumption of ASP in recent years (Table 7-1) was detailed in Chapters 7 and 8. About 5,000 different products now contain aspartame. *Currently, an estimated 54 percent of adults in the United States consume them!* I have underscored the potential public health hazards resulting from the lack of adequate evaluation of ASP in humans by corporate-neutral investigators prior to Food and Drug Administration (FDA) approval in spite of considerable troubling data (Roberts 1987b, 1988d,e, 1989a, 1992b).

Personal Observations on Aspartame Reactors

Severe confusion, gross impairment of memory, or both, were reported by 28.5% of the first 551 reactors to ASP products in my series (Roberts 1988e, 1989a, 1991a, 1992b). The majority were 20-59 years, averaging 45 years in age. The breakdown by age groups was as follows:

10 - 19 years	3.9%
20 - 29 years	13.7%
30 - 39 years	25.5%
40 - 49 years	22.5%
50 - 59 years	17.6%
60 - 69 years	16.7%

Two aspects demonstrate convincingly the causative role of aspartame-containing products in patient reactions. First, there was marked improvement or disappearance of the confusion and memory loss after ASP products were avoided. Second, these symptoms promptly and predictably recurred on rechallenge.

Most persons so afflicted had consumed modest to large amounts of ASP products in many commercially-available forms—especially "diet" beverages (averaging 16 mg/oz), and a popular tabletop sweetener (averaging 35 mg/packet). However, even relatively small amounts of ASP could induce confusion and memory impairment. This was particularly impressive in the case of diet sodas that probably had been stored for many months, or when this sweetener was added to hot beverages.

- A 31-year-old nurse with a prior ASP-associated convulsion became confused and "very incoherent" the morning after drinking three sips of an ASP-containing beverage initially thought to be a "regular" soda.

- A 61-year-old executive bought a light snack and coffee at a fast food outlet before playing golf. Because the saccharin sweetener he used was not stocked, he used an ASP tabletop sweetener. He became confused and behaved erratically on the golf course. His memory cleared within two hours, with no recollection of this episode. He then recalled two comparable episodes after drinking ASP-sweetened coffee at the homes of friends. There was no recurrence after abstaining from ASP products.

Several findings in my database of reactors to ASP products (currently numbering over 640) are germane:

- A 3:1 female preponderance was consistently encountered. The apparent higher incidence of AD among women in many studies (Chapter 16) is pertinent.

- An impressive familial incidence, averaging 22 percent, was found (Roberts 1988e, 1989a, 1989b). Furthermore, multiple family members often evidenced similar types of reactions.

- Many patients volunteered their fear of having "early Alzheimer's disease" before a reaction to ASP products was diagnosed. Most felt relieved and reassured when their confusion, memory loss, and other neuropsychiatric features subsided after avoiding such products once this diagnosis had been made.

These observations have been independently confirmed by the FDA from its file of complaint letters. Numerous consumers voluntarily reported comparable confusion and memory loss associated with the use of ASP (Tollefson 1987). Over half the complainants were between 20 and 59 years of age; about 85% were female.

Some astute correspondents have projected the public health problems associated with such induced confusion and memory loss, based on their own reactions to aspartame products. For example, an attorney wrote: "I can't help but wonder how many other people are being injured by cognitive impairment from aspartame without even realizing what is happening to them."

Typical Reactions

ASP-associated confusion and memory loss ranged from subtle "forgettings" and "difficulty in concentrating" to gross intellectual incapacitation. Some examples:

- A 30-year-old female sales consultant noted, "I could not consciously remember what I had done or said."
- An engineer had trouble remembering "names and descriptive adjectives."
- Several persons confided that they occasionally couldn't remember their own names when using ASP products.
- A 64-year-old building inspector volunteered, "I could not think straight."
- An 18-year-old male forgot where he was or where to turn when driving in his neighborhood while drinking two liters of ASP-containing soft drinks daily.
- A 47-year-old woman expressed extreme concern over the striking deterioration of her prized "photographic memory" when consuming ASP products.
- Experienced secretaries described many typing and computer errors after using ASP products.
- A 34-year-old English and Spanish instructor "began having trouble sequencing assignments" when she drank two cans of diet cola daily.
- A 52-year-old executive complained of difficulty in remembering whom he was calling after dialing a number, and expressed concern over incipient Alzheimer's disease. The problem disappeared when he avoided ASP products.
- A 58-year-old man complained that his memory had become "so bad that if I am cooking something in the kitchen, I'm likely to forget about it." There was concomitant headache, dizziness, decreased vision and depression. These symptoms disappeared one week after discontinuing ASP beverages, and did not recur over the ensuing two years.
- A colleague in Phoenix told me about a young female patient who had been consuming a six-pack of aspartame sodas daily to lose weight. Finding herself "lost" in a food market, she searched through her purse to get help. She finally located her husband's office phone number, and was able to contact him. The confusion did not recur when she avoided aspartame products.

Dr. Nicholas Petkas, a medical colleague, depicted the "aging" effects of ASP products in a cartoon (Figure 9-2).

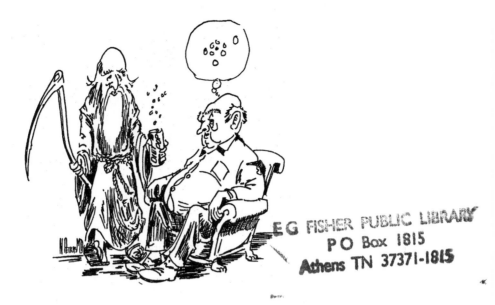

Figure 9-2

Underlying Mechanisms

The confusion and memory loss associated with use of ASP products probably reflect multiple mechanisms. They include the following:

- Unchecked flooding of the brain by L-phenylalanine, L-aspartic acid, and their L-iso or D-stereoisomers (Chapter 7)

- The toxic effects of free methyl alcohol

- Metabolic breakdown products of ASP formed during heating and prolonged storage (i.e., more than two months)

- Binding of excitatory amino acids to the membranes of brain cells

- Dysfunction induced by amino acid-derived neurotransmitters and related substances (Chapter 5)

- Induced or aggravated hypoglycemia (Chapter 8) due to excessive insulin secretion (Melchior 1991)

- A marked increase of beta-endorphins (Melchior 1991)

Phenylalanine. Phenylalanine is unique in terms of brain metabolism and neurotransmitter function. It has the highest affinity for crossing the blood-brain barrier of all the circulating amino acids. Furthermore, the exit time required for brain levels to decrease by half is longer for phenylalanine than for several other amino acids (Lajtha 1962).

There are other evidences for the uniqueness of phenylalanine.

- Dietary carbohydrate does not decrease its absorption, as is the case when leucine (another amino acid) is ingested (Krempf 1993).

- Roznoski, Huang, and Burns (1993) studied the effects of phenylalanine on the peripheral and central kinetics and metabolism of L-dopa in monkeys. Phenylalanine appears to inhibit the transport of L-dopa into cells, its

81

metabolism within cells, or both.

Aspartic Acid. Aspartic acid is present throughout the brain. It can exert a strong excitatory effect comparable to glutamate (see above). These aspects of its metabolism are noteworthy:

- As a free amino acid, aspartic acid is absorbed through an active transport system. This contrasts with peptides containing aspartic acid.

- Aspartic acid is rapidly converted to aspartate and glutamate, as evidenced by the significant elevation of both aspartate and glutamate after ingesting a loading dose. It is then transported across both nerve membranes and the blood-brain barrier.

- In experimental studies, insulin-induced hypoglycemia (Chapter 8) causes a sharp increase of brain aspartate concentrations (Chapman 1987). By contrast, glutamate and glutamine levels decline.

The experimental administration of L-aspartic acid can induce changes within the hypothalamus, especially in susceptible young animals. Later, they develop obesity, skeletal stunting, and reduced reproductive-organ size. Injected into the brain, both aspartic acid and its N-methyl-D-aspartate derivatives are powerful convulsants (Turski 1984).

Stereoisomers (Mirror Images) and Other Metabolites of Aspartic Acid. The conversion (racemization) of amino acids tends to proceed from the biologically common L (levo) configuration to the uncommon D (dextro) configuration (Chapter 7). D-aspartic acid and other racemate metabolites increase in ASP products during excessive heat or prolonged storage (Boehm 1984).

The accumulation of D-aspartic acid in the brain with aging has considerable significance. Man et al (1987b) reported that its presence in the white matter of the human brain increases considerably from infancy to about 35 years. They suggested that _such increased D-aspartate levels could lead to changes in protein configuration and associated dysfunction._

Clinical Perspectives

The observations cited require that persons who develop otherwise-unexplained confusion and memory loss, regardless of age, be queried about the consumption of aspartame products. Also, they should be observed at least one month after avoiding such products before being subjected to extensive neurologic testing. Ensuing dramatic improvement could spare them the onus of being misdiagnosed as having probable Alzheimer's disease.

Similar considerations apply to the intake of other phenylalanine products and amino acid preparations. Most no longer can be purchased over the counter in Canada. (Canada instituted this policy after the profound effects of such products on brain function were recognized.)

Insights Concerning Alzheimer's Disease

The foregoing discussion of some adverse effects of aspartame and its breakdown products on brain function clarifies a number of observations that pertain to AD. Although technical, interested readers may wish a summary of these details.

Aspartate metabolism is altered in AD.

- A significant amount of aspartic acid exists in the amyloid precursor protein (APP) of brain amyloid (Chapter 4).

- Aspartate binding is reduced in the cerebral cortex of AD brains (Cross 1987).

- The uptake and binding of D-aspartic acid appears to be impaired *early* in AD brain cells (Procter 1988).

- The increase of D-aspartate and beta-linked L-isoaspartate in AD neurofibrillary tangles (Schapira 1987, Payan 1992) is extraordinary. There are 1.5-2 times more total defective aspartate in AD neurofibrillary tangles—most as the beta-linked L-isoaspartate.

- In a patient with late-onset AD, Peacock et al (1993) found a novel mutation in codon 665 wherein aspartate was substituted for glutamine.

Aluminum (Chapter 10) increases the conversion of aspartic acid to D-aspartate in living brain protein. This could have a bearing upon the increased amounts of D-aspartate and L-isoaspartate present in neurofibrillary tangles.

The contributory role of phenylalanine (PHE) requires much study. For example, a *single* amino acid mutation—involving the substitution of phenylalanine for valine in amyloid precursor protein—appears to be the basis for at least one type of hereditary AD (Murrell 1991).

Another remarkable coincidence is the presence of aspartic acid next to phenylalanine in cholecystokinin (CCK). CCK is a neuropeptide that plays a significant role in learning, memory, behavior, and acetylcholine release.

- The amino acid sequence (using conventional abbreviations) of its biologically active form is ASP-TYR (SO3H)-MET-GLY-TRP-MET-*ASP-PHE*-NH2 (Brownstein 1985).

- CCK exists in unusually high concentrations within the cerebral cortex, the hippocampus (Chapter 4), and related areas (Crawley 1985).

- CCK meets most of the criteria for a neurotransmitter—namely, its presence in nerve tissue, its localization in neurons, its concentration in synaptic vesicles, and its release by specific stimuli (Goltermann 1985).

The amino acid sequence of cholecystokinin and its documented biological effects could explain some of the cerebral and metabolic reactions to products containing aspartame (Roberts 1989a, 1992b).

- CCK may cause or exaggerate glucose depletion in the brain. Tamminga et al (1985) reported that the peripheral administration of CCK-8 decreases glucose utilization in certain pertinent areas.

- The magnitude of weight loss has been dramatic among some persons using aspartame products. Rogers, Keedwell and Blundell (1991) suggested that aspartame inhibits food intake in humans because it is a cholecystokinin releaser.

ALCOHOL

Experienced neurologists and psychiatrists recognize the extraordinary neurotoxicity of ethyl alcohol, especially when chronically abused. Alcohol also is known to alter the blood-brain barrier (Lee 1962), thereby exposing the hippocampus and related structures vital for memory to this and other neurotoxins.

The adverse effects of alcohol include atrophy of the brain in young alcoholics, a phenomenon clearly demonstrable by imaging studies.

Associated nutritional disorders in alcoholics can alter brain function. They might be prevented by dietary supplementation (Chapter 18), and insistence upon frequent feedings to counter alcohol-induced hypoglycemia (Chapter 8).

DIETARY NEUROTOXINS IN HEREDITARY DISORDERS

There are relatively large numbers of "carriers" or "heterozygotes" for important hereditary metabolic diseases within the general population. In the present context, the carrier state refers to difficulty handling common foods or their breakdown products, which then can accumulate and damage the nervous system. These problems have been made more complex by "advances" in food technology.

This discussion will be limited to phenylketonuria, galactosemia and lactase deficiency.

I. Phenylketonuria

About one out of 50 persons in the general population is a phenylketonuria (PKU) carrier. Individuals with this disorder are unable to handle phenylalanine because phenylalanine hydroxylase, the enzyme required for its metabolism, is absent or deficient.

The hazards to PKU heterozygotes from ingesting phenylalanine in food, food additives (e.g., aspartame), and other products are well known. They include neuropsychiatric, metabolic, ocular and developmental problems. The neurotoxic effects of phenylalanine and its stereoisomers were reviewed above.

An ongoing threat of neurologic damage exists even when PKU was effectively treated early in life by dietary avoidance. Indeed, affected persons must remain watchful for the rest of their lives. They may not realize the threat of certain products that contain phenylalanine, notwithstanding some related statement on the labels of aspartame products.

> Thompson et al (1991) studied 26 PKU patients who had achieved blood phenylalanine concentrations within the desired therapeutic range during their first eight years. Although none evidenced gross neurologic dysfunction, definite abnormalities could be found in 23 by magnetic resonance imaging (MRI) studies.

II. Galactosemia

Galactosemia results from three inherited disorders involving the metabolism of

84

galactose, a simple sugar. Herman M. Kalckar (1965), Professor of Biochemical Chemistry at Harvard Medical School, referred to galactose as "one of the freaks of evolution."

This genetic disorder reflects a deficiency of the several enzymes required to convert galactose to glucose in cells. About one percent of the population are heterozygotes for the classic galactosemia trait (Segal 1989). It is three times more frequent in certain groups, notably blacks and Italians.

The adverse effects of galactose accumulation include failure to thrive, mental retardation, cataracts, blindness, liver disease, infertility, premature menopause, and severe neurologic disorders such as tremors and seizures.

Galactose intolerance is pertinent to this discussion for several reasons:

- Galactose toxicity can be demonstrated in tissue culture.

- Rodents that are fed galactose-enriched diets develop neural dysfunction and early vascular structural changes identical to those in diabetic animals (Williamson 1993).

- Persons who are prone to reactive hypoglycemia (Chapter 8) risk severe attacks after ingesting galactose because it stimulates the release of insulin.

- Although galactosemic children are able to survive to adulthood by adhering to galactose-free diets, late-onset neurologic and other complications can be anticipated (Friedman 1989).

- It was formerly thought that dairy products were the principal foods containing appreciable galactose. Recent research indicates its presence in others. Galactosemics may not realize the galactose content of many commonly consumed fruits and vegetables, some of which contain over 10 mg galactose per 100 gm—e.g., dates; papaya; bell peppers; tomato; watermelon (Gross 1991).

- Novel food formulations containing galactose have been approved without extensive pre-marketing trials on humans. For example, more non-fat milk is being added to fat-reduced dairy products. Similarly, NutraSweet BulkFree® is produced by combining milk solids nonfat (MSNF) with lactase, an enzyme that cleaves lactose into glucose and galactose (discussed below).

III. Lactose Intolerance

Intolerance to lactose or "milk sugar" is largely due to the lack of lactase, an intestinal enzyme. It is *common* among virtually all populations except persons of Northern European origin. Indeed, lactose-tolerant individuals constitute a small minority of the world's population.

Although usually hereditary, this deficiency may be acquired from changes in the intestinal wall due to disease.

The associated symptoms of gas and indigestion can be relieved by adding various beta-galactosidases that lower lactose concentrations in milk. For example, LactAid® is derived from the yeast *Kluyveromyces lactis.* Milk in fermented form—such as cheese, yogurt and buttermilk—also may be tolerated.

The potential long-term effects of increased galactose intake, as well as its absorption from lactose-hydrolyzed milk, are not fully understood, especially relative to central nervous system dysfunction.

10

THE ROLE OF ALUMINUM

*Few subjects cause greater controversy than the assessment
of the potential health hazard of a chemical. The more
widely the chemical is used, the greater will be the
potential impact on public health and the
subsequent scatter of opinions and
attitudes. Often, these opinions are
impossible to equate.**

D. D. Bryson (1981)

*The chemicals we ingest may affect more than our own health.
They affect the health and vitality of future generations.
The danger is that many of these chemicals
may not harm us, but will later do
silent violence to our children.*

Senator Abraham S. Ribicoff (1971)

    The presence of aluminum within the brain changes that characterize Alzheimer's disease (AD) requires analysis of its role relative to causation. Although aluminum has been referred to as a "dementing ion," its relevance to AD remains controversial. For example, one argument advanced by the aluminum industry concerning an inferred relationship between aluminum in tap water and the increased incidence of AD in certain areas (e.g., Scotland) is the local clustering of many relatives with familial AD.

---

*©1981 *The Lancet.* Reproduced with permission.

86

Candy et al (1986) identified aluminosilicates within the core of AD plaques (Chapter 4), and suggested that aluminosilicates "may be involved in the initiation or early stages of senile plaque formation." These and other insights provide a basis for certain precautions and recommendations aimed at preventing AD (Chapter 17).

PERSPECTIVES

Aluminum is the third most abundant metal in the earth's crust. Yet, no physiological role has been ascribed to it.

More than twice the amount of aluminum now exists in the body (0.9 parts per million or ppm) than in our ancestors (0.4 ppm).

The widespread use of aluminum ranks it among the foremost industrial innovations and ecologic changes of this era. In keeping with the writer's premise that AD is a "disease of the 20th Century," aluminum was not previously used in any foods or drugs. (The Hall process for manufacturing aluminum from bauxite ore began in the 1890s—about 15 years before Alzheimer described his case.) Aluminum is present in cans, cookware, aluminum foil, toiletries, medications and drinking water.

Aluminum production continues to increase annually in the United States. By 1991, it was estimated at 4,164,768 metric tons (*The Wall Street Journal* August 20, 1991, p. A-1). Demand rose in the United States by nine percent during the first eight months of 1993, coupled with a "tidal wave" of exports from Russia and other former Soviet republics (Aeppel 1993).

> There is greater demand of aluminum by the automotive industry as a substitute for steel. Its expanded uses include wheels, bumper systems, door intrusion beams, sunroof tracks and car frames.

Public health authorities generally place the maximum safe intake of aluminum at 3 milligrams (mg) daily. This amount is readily exceeded. Some examples:

- Aluminum increases 75-fold in water heated to 88 degrees C in an aluminum pot. This level represents more than 30 times the recommended limit of 50 micrograms (μg)/liter (Jackson 1989).

- A single antacid tablet may contain 50 mg or more of an aluminum compound. Accordingly, more than 1,000 mg (!) could be consumed daily in treating common disorders of the esophagus and stomach with average recommended doses.

There is no unanimous agreement that aluminum intake causes AD. Some even regard its presence in AD lesions as a coincidental artifact. However, the considerable body of evidence for aluminum neurotoxicity, and its ability to reinforce other neurotoxic influences (Chapters 9 and 11), cannot be ignored. There is more convincing evidence for the presence of aluminum in neurofibrillary tangle-bearing neurons than in the early neuritic plaques (Peri 1980).

ALUMINUM AND ALZHEIMER'S DISEASE

Four independent arguments support the concept that aluminum intake contributes to the evolution of AD (Andrews 1991).

- Multiple epidemiologic studies demonstrate an association between bioavailable aluminum in drinking water and the incidence of AD (see below).

- Aluminum can alter the physiological function of neurons even when there are no demonstrable changes in them. It may play a pivotal role in AD by increasing oxidative stress on nerve cells.
- Aluminum disturbs over 60 neurochemical reactions at concentrations likely to exist in the human brain.
- The clinical progression of AD appears to be slowed by desferrioxamine (Crapper-McLachlan 1991). This trivalent metal chelator is capable of removing aluminum from the AD brain.

Excess amounts of aluminum have been found by various methods—notably, scanning electron microscopy and x-ray spectrometry—in both amyloid plaques and neurofibrillary tangles (Candy 1986, Crapper 1980). The latter may contain three to four times more aluminum than healthy neurons. Some contend that aluminum accumulates in the AD brain because it binds to defective beta and tau proteins, which are more fundamentally involved with the disease process.

Aluminum also collects on the DNA of strategic brain cell nuclei. Any damage inflicted on these nuclei is therefore likely to affect memory and behavior.

ALUMINUM INTAKE

The daily intake of aluminum from all sources by persons in the United States is estimated at 20 to 40 mg, compared to the maximum safe amount of 3 mg. The sources include foods, water, aluminum cookware, and others mentioned below.

Excessive aluminum has been detected in drinking water (Martyn 1989, Powell 1990), infant formulas (Bishop 1989, Fisher 1989), dolomite and bone meal (Roberts 1981a,b; 1983), most antacids (further discussed below), and other commonly used products.

- Davenport and Goodall (1992) found aluminum in orange juice. This probably occurred during processing with contaminated tap water used for its reconstitution.

- High levels of aluminum are present in foods processed with aluminum products. They include baking powder (e.g., chocolate cake and waffles), aluminum calcium sulfate (as an anti-caking agent), aluminum potassium sulfate and aluminum sodium sulfate (as firming agents, and as carriers for bleaching agents in cereal flours and some cheeses), and aluminum stearate (as a defoaming agent).

- Considerable aluminum may be consumed in tea (Coriat 1986). The tea plant (Camellia sinensis) concentrates the aluminum absorbed from acid soil into its leaves. Black tea contains 500-1500 mg Al/kg; the prepared beverage contains 2-6 mg/liter (L). A recent national study of AD in Canada suggests that patients with this disease were 2-1/2 times more likely to be tea drinkers—defined as consuming at least one cup a day (*The Calgary Sun* May 7, 1993, p. 26).

- <u>Many drugs, cosmetics, antiperspirants and deodorants</u> contain aluminum compounds, which render them smooth, creamy and pourable.

Drinking Water

Current public health policies generally recommend that (1) the aluminum concentration of drinking water be reduced to 50 µg/L for short-term use, and 10 µg/L for long-term use, and (2) the total amount ingested not exceed 3 mg daily (*The Lancet* 1992; 339:713-714).

Several studies have impressively linked AD with the ingestion of excessive aluminum in drinking water supplies.

- Analysis of its concentration at nine catchment areas in Britain revealed a 1.7-fold incidence of AD among populations that drank water containing 1-10 µg aluminum per liter.

- Martyn et al (1989) reported the incidence of AD to be 1.5 times higher in districts of England and Wales where the aluminum concentration in drinking water exceeded 0.11 mg/L than where the concentration was below 0.01 mg/L.

- Neri and Hewitt (1991) implicated the aluminum consumed in drinking water as a factor contributing to AD. They correlated the diagnosis of AD or presenile dementia in 2344 patients, aged 55 or older, with concentrations of aluminum content in the drinking water. (Reliable water quality data were available through the Water Quality Surveillance Programme of the Ontario Ministry of the Environment.) An unbroken rising sequence—with aluminum concentrations from below 0.1 mg/L to above 0.2 mg/L—indicated such relative risk.

- A similar 30-year follow-up study of 2,000 males in the Ontario Longitudinal Study of Aging (Forbes 1991) is noteworthy. It revealed that men were three times more likely to develop some form of mental impairment in areas where the aluminum concentration was high.

- Forbes and McAnley (1992) reported an odds ratio of 1.86 for older persons having symptoms of impaired mental functioning who drank water with a high aluminum concentration.

Aluminum Containers

Juices, soft drinks, beer and other beverages are packaged in aluminum cans. Such use is enormous and increases during warm weather (*The Wall Street Journal* July 1, 1991, p. B-4A).

- Soft drinks can contain up to 3.9 mg per can.
- The aluminum content of non-cola drinks is almost six times higher in cans than in bottles, and nearly three times higher for cola beverages in cans than in bottles (Duggan 1992).

Antacids

Most conventional antacids contain considerable amounts of aluminum compounds (Robertson 1989, Withers 1989, Salusky 1991). Sucralfate (Carafate®), a drug widely used to treat peptic ulcer by protecting the stomach's lining, contains eight aluminum and sulfate molecules attached to a sucrose nucleus. The recommended dosage is one gram (containing about 200 mg aluminum), taken four times daily on an empty stomach.

Infants with normal kidney function who received aluminum-containing antacids for one week or longer were found to have markedly elevated plasma aluminum levels (Tsou 1991).

In another study utilizing atomic absorption spectroscopy, Kisters et al (1990) found elevated aluminum concentrations both in the blood plasma and in the gastric mucous membrane of individuals who had ingested aluminum-containing antacids for two weeks.

Aluminum Antiperspirants and Deodorants

A case-control study in the State of Washington showed a significant association (odds ratio of 1.6) between AD and the prior use of aluminum-containing antiperspirants (Graves 1990).

"Dialysis Dementia"

Aluminum neurotoxicity probably accounts for "dialysis dementia." This term signifies neurological deterioration of uremic patients on long-term hemodialysis (Salusky 1991). The large amount of aluminum present in the brain is attributed to its absorption from ingested phosphate-binding gels that contain aluminum, and aluminum in the water used to prepare the dialysis fluid.

Industrial Waste

Industrial waste constitutes another potential source of environmental exposure to considerable amounts of aluminum.

- Severe neurologic changes were exhibited by 25 workers at an aluminum smelting plant (White 1992). Their symptoms included loss of balance, poor memory, impaired abstract reasoning and depression. Three-fourths of the workers evidenced impairment in memory tests.

- A similar syndrome is known as potroem palsy. (The term refers to the reduction of aluminum manufactured in steel pots.)

- Sanz et al (1992) reported two children with excess aluminum attributed to the polluted environment of their neighborhood from a factory where aluminum was recycled.

FACTORS INFLUENCING ALUMINUM ABSORPTION AND TRANSPORT

Physical, environmental and medical factors can influence the gastrointestinal

90

absorption of aluminum. Some may represent avoidable risks (Chapter 17).

- Aluminum in more available in <u>drinking water</u> than in foods and antacids.
- Aluminum absorption increases with <u>acidity</u>, as when it is ingested with citric acid. Lemon and other citrus juices tend to enhance the absorption of aluminum (Butterworth 1992).
- <u>Ascorbic acid</u> (vitamin C) augments aluminum absorption and increases aluminum concentrations in the blood, liver, brain and bone (Domingo 1991).
- Certain <u>aluminum salts</u> (aluminum hydroxide; aluminum citrates) are readily more absorbed.
- Some <u>lipid-soluble aluminum complexes</u> (e.g., the aluminum maltol present in instant chocolate mixes) are absorbed.
- Aluminum absorption increases dramatically with <u>impaired kidney function</u> and during prolonged <u>total intravenous alimentation</u>.
- The brain is more susceptible to aluminum intoxication during <u>pregnancy, infancy and childhood.</u>

The Influences of Other Elements

Fluoride. Fluoride is generally considered protective against aluminum absorption. However, the leaching of aluminum from utensils might be increased by trace quantities of fluoride (Tennakone 1987a), perhaps because fluoride ions tend to disrupt the protective film of aluminum oxide.

In relevant experimental studies, the drinking water of rats was dosed with graduated levels of aluminum <u>and</u> fluoride. Behavioral changes were noted after 45 to 50 weeks, coupled with loss of brain cells within the neocortex and hippocampus (Isaacson 1992).

Calcium and Magnesium. The role of aluminum in the amyotrophic lateral sclerosis-parkinsonism-dementia syndrome among Guamanian Chamorros has been investigated. A large amount was found in the drinking water and garden soils of Guam, along with unusually low levels of calcium and magnesium (Perl 1982). This combination appears to favor aberrations of mineral metabolism that could enhance aluminum deposition within the central nervous system.

The reduction of magnesium in AD brain cells interferes with energy availability, and increases free radical formation and vulnerability to excitotoxins.

Silicon. An inverse relation has been demonstrated between aluminum and silicon in water supplies (Edwardson 1993). This suggests that dissolved silicon could be an important factor in limiting the absorption of dietary aluminum. Birchall (1993) subsequently suggested cooking in silicic-acid-rich water, or the co-consumption of such water or food enriched with silicon to restrict the absorption of aluminum present in food.

Transport Mechanisms

Circulating aluminum is carried by transferrin. This iron-binding protein tends to be transported across the blood-brain barrier (Chapter 11) to sites where transferrin receptors are the highest—notably, the cortex, hippocampus, septum and amygdala.

These structures also are the preferential locations for most AD plaques (McGregor 1991).

Aluminum penetrates red blood cells in the presence of increased circulating sodium L-glutamate, an amino-acid neurotoxin (Chapter 9). Rat studies indicate that an aluminum glutamate complex can pass through the blood-brain barrier, and then be deposited in the brain.

MECHANISMS OF ALUMINUM NEUROTOXICITY

Aluminum can damage the brain directly and indirectly in various ways. Its effects on brain metabolism, glucose utilization, brain cell nuclei, receptor channels, the blood-brain barrier, and aspartic acid stereoisomers will be briefly considered. Aluminum also impairs the uptake of choline (Chapter 5), and interacts with iron (Chapter 11).

Effects of Aluminum on Brain Metabolism

Aluminum inhibits important enzymes that perform essential metabolic processes. They include cyclic adenosine monophosphate (AMP), adenylate cyclase, and phospho-diesterase activities (Jaouni 1985).

The unique property of aluminum as a crosslinker contributes to the formation of neurofibrillary tangles and their precursors (Bjorksten 1991). (Crosslinkers are chemical compounds having two or more reactive points capable of forming strong chemical bonds between two larger molecules, and binding them together. Small amounts of a crosslinking molecule therefore can effect great change).

The direct neurotoxic effects of aluminum have been studied experimentally by Dr. Jonathan J. Lipman (1988, 1989). The delivery of aluminum directly to the brain induced behavioral abnormalities, learning and memory derangements, and electroencephalographic changes.

Effects of Aluminum on Glucose Utilization

Lipman et al (1988, 1989) noted a *significant decrease in the brain's ability to metabolize glucose after exposure to aluminum*. Aluminum inhibits hexokinase in the brain, and competes with magnesium in adenosine triphosphate (ATP)-related energy release (Lipman 1989a).

Increased aluminum deposition also can aggravate cerebral glucopenia (Chapter 8). Ribak et al (1989) demonstrated this phenomenon and ensuing epilepsy after implanting aluminum gel in monkeys.

Effects of Aluminum On Nuclei of Brain Cells

By interacting with nucleic acid polyphosphates, aluminum damages chromatin… thereby altering DNA synthesis and replication (Lukiw 1989).

Effects of Aluminum on the N-Methyl-D-Aspartate Receptor Channel

Aluminum disrupts the magnesium block of the N-methyl-D-aspartate (NMDA) receptor channel in central nervous system neurons. Uncontrolled activation of excitatory synapses ensues, with ensuing calcium influx and cell death (Brenner 1989).

Effects of Aluminum on the Blood-Brain Barrier

Aluminum alters the permeability of the vital blood-brain barrier (Chapter 11). It thereby makes the brain more vulnerable for access by potentially neurotoxic amino acids, small peptides (such as beta-endorphin), hormones, toxins and drugs (Banks 1983, 1989).

Effects of Aluminum on Aspartic Acid Stereoisomers

Aluminum combines with (chelates) aspartic acid. This tends to accelerate the conversion (racemization) of L-aspartic acid to its "mirror images" (Chapter 9) in living brain protein.

Anderson et al (1990) fed supplementary aluminum salts to rats for ten weeks. Their brains accumulated 65 to 182 percent excess aluminum, compared to controls. There was a concomitant increase of D-aspartate levels in brain tissue. Such accelerated amino acid racemization to the abnormal D-stereoisomer (Chapter 7) has considerable significance in view of the increased amounts of D-aspartate and L-isoasparate demonstrated in AD neurofibrillary tangles (Chapters 4).

11

THE ROLE OF OTHER ENVIRONMENTAL NEUROTOXINS IN AIR, WATER, FOOD AND DRUGS

Thou speaks't like a physician, Helicanus, That ministers a potion unto me That thou wouldst tremble to receive thyself.

Shakespeare
(*Pericles, Prince of Tyre* Act I, Scene 2)

There is no "mass hysteria" or "chemophobia." There is growing awareness of the preciousness of human life, the banal nature of much of what industry is producing, and the gross inadequacy of efforts to protect the public from long-term chemical hazards.*

Earon S. Davis (1989)

FDA's goal is simple: We want people to have access to products that are safe, and we want to assure consumers that claims made about the health and nutritional benefits are truthful... but hype cannot overwhelm science.

Dr. David Kessler (1993)
(FDA Commissioner)

---

*©Reproduced with permission of Earon S. Davis, M.P.H.

94

The general public is exposed to many neurotoxic substances that can cause severe brain injury. They include drugs, food additives (MSG; aspartame), carbon monoxide, certain metals (mercury; aluminum; lead; arsenic), pesticides, and other chemicals.

A sobering evidence for the persistent—and increasing—threat of chemical pollution is disclosure by the Du Pont Company that its toxic chemical releases increased six percent in 1991 to 233.3 million pounds (*The Wall Street Journal* May 19, 1993, p. B-4). A considerable amount involved the pumping of more chemical byproducts into deep injection wells. In view of the neurotoxicity of iron (see below), the large quantity of ferric chloride therein is noteworthy.

Numerous studies concerning the ongoing contamination of food and water stress full accountability for the eventual effects of adding potentially dangerous substances to soil, water, animal feed or processed foods—whether as pesticides, additives, hormones or radiation.

The fact that greater exposure to neurotoxins preceded or paralleled the dramatic rise of Alzheimer's disease (AD) since the mid-20th Century suggests their role as significant "risk factors." This idea is reinforced by the observation that stimulation of amyloid precursor protein (APP), with subsequent deposition of beta-amyloid (Chapter 4), represents a response by many tissues to injury—including exposure to toxic chemicals, both organic and inorganic (Regland 1992). In turn, beta-amyloid can enhance the degeneration induced by excitotoxins such as glutamate and related amino acids (Choi 1992).

Neurotoxins: At Home and The Workplace is a report of hearings conducted in June 1986 by the Committee on Science and Technology, U.S. House of Representatives. The book, later issued by the U.S. Government Printing Office (1989), defines neurotoxins as "chemicals that poison the nervous system." The introductory statement began:

"Millions of people are exposed every day to neurotoxic industrial chemicals, including solvents, pesticides, drugs, food additives and cosmetics. People who have experienced acute exposure to neurotoxins show the readily recognizable symptoms of dizziness, nausea, muscle weakness, and blurred vision. But symptoms of chronic exposure—such as increased irritability, *loss of memory, inability to concentrate,* and sexual dysfunction—may go unnoticed, or be ascribed to social pressures rather than to neurological damage." (My italics for emphasis)

An "industrial river" with input from industry, agriculture and community waste can contain as many as 200 chemicals This poses a potentially enormous problem in terms of neurotoxicity and cancer for the consumers of drinking water derived from the treatment of these waterways. Both the frequency and quality of state inspections have come under considerable criticism, especially when gross deficiencies resulted in severe medical disease. For example, cross-connections have allowed both sewage and industrial pollutants to leak into pipes transmitting drinking water. The use of filters to trap contaminants becomes less effective if they are not serviced at the recommended frequency (e.g., changing carbon filters every four to six months).

Concern over neurotoxicity has increased with the awareness that *an estimated 70,000 chemicals in commercial use have not yet been tested for adverse neurological effects* (Stone 1993). The EPA has attempted to address this deficiency by incorporating assays for neurotoxicity in the batteries of animal tests used to assess the potential health effects of commercial chemicals. One measures the levels in brain of a protein called glial fibrillary acidic protein (GFAP), which can detect damage missed by standard microscopic screens (Stone 1993).

Exposure to exogenous neurotoxins early in life can have profound long-term effects. Lead provides a classic example. Another is the since-discontinued incorporation of monosodium glutamate (MSG) and hydrolyzed vegetable protein (HVP) in commercial baby foods (Chapter 9). The induction of disease by some environmental factor also may be influenced by one's genetic predisposition (Chapter 3).

Cognitive impairment may occur in children who were exposed <u>prenatally</u> to chemicals and neurotoxins. In Yu-Cheng ("oil disease"), for example, the mothers of Taiwanese children so afflicted had been exposed to high levels of heat-degraded polychlorinated biphenyls (PCBs) (Chen 1992).

The extraordinary prevalence and magnitude of <u>perinatal</u> exposures to licit and illicit drugs, alcohol and tobacco have enormous implications relative to neurobehavioral dysfunction. Vega et al (1993) reported exposure to drugs and alcohol in 11.35 percent of maternity patients at California hospitals in 1992 (about 67,000 women); 52,346 reported exposures to tobacco. Similarly, 12.1 percent of women in South Carolina who gave birth used drugs or alcohol (based on urine testing) according to a 1991 report by the South Carolina Commission on Alcohol and Drug Abuse.

Clinicians should be alerted to <u>additional manifestations of toxin-induced injury</u> in tissues other than the brain. They might include infertility due to dramatically lessened sperm counts, and the loss of hair or teeth. Further research will be required to establish the validity of such correlates with nerve cell destruction.

Some frequent sources of chemical contamination and mold-mildew development in homes, along with preventive measures, are listed in Chapter 17.

The Blood-Brain Barrier

There is considerable evidence that the blood-brain barrier is meant to serve as a protective mechanism for keeping neurotoxins out of the brain. This barrier resides chiefly in the "tight junctions" of brain capillaries. Its development during the first trimester of pregnancy indicates the importance of such a protective mechanism.

The blood-brain barrier has been described as both a "chemical filter" and a "biogenic wall." It is probably altered by aspartame, aspartame breakdown products, and monosodium glutamate (Chapter 9).

Obstacles

Any regimen aimed at preventing Alzheimer's disease will require both the avoidance and reduction of environmental neurotoxins. This is the basis for an escalating "detox" movement, especially in the home environment.

Unfortunately, the success of efforts aimed at reducing chemical exposure continues to be thwarted by numerous obstacles from industry, government, and even the health professions. Hence, prevention is left primarily to concerned individuals, especially parents.

- Companies that produced and transported large quantities of hazardous waste (at least 2,200 pounds monthly) more than doubled in Florida over a seven-year period (*The Miami Herald* November 24, 1992, p. B-5). At the same time, state inspections dwindled to only 1.2 percent of those producers. Furthermore, 25 percent of violators (including boat manufacturers, auto painting and body repair shops, and furniture refinishers) failed to correct their operations—e.g., the improper labeling of hazardous waste drums; disposing waste at nonregulated facilities.

- Awareness of the long atmospheric life of many halogenated chemicals indicates the need for extreme care before approving them. Ravishankara et al (1993) reported that the lifetimes of fluorinated gases can range from 300 to 2,000 years!

Clinicians who must deal with suspected neurotoxic illness will find that the literature on neurotoxins is largely useless. As a rule, one cannot rely on the laboratory to detect neurotoxin effects, especially from prolonged and low-level exposure. Moreover, corporate-funded testing is often tantamount to "kill and count them."

"Preemptive science" has caused our society to suffer enormously when it enabled the introduction and prolonged use of neurotoxic additives and other substances. Even though some were subsequently withdrawn, much harm had been incurred during the intervening extended period of evaluation for safety, then followed by delaying legal maneuvers.

In this regard, the Generally Recognized As Safe (GRAS) designation has contributed to considerable misery. Such a designation should not have been condoned when enough reasonable doubt existed about a product to warrant further careful research before it was permitted to enter the food supply or environment.

NEUROTOXIC ELEMENTS

A number of mineral elements have neurotoxic effects that may initiate or compound the pathologic changes of neurodegenerative disorders such as AD and Parkinson's disease. Aluminum neurotoxicity was considered in Chapter 10.

> Gorell et al (1991) analyzed the death rates in Michigan for persons with Parkinson's disease in terms of exposure to various metals—viz., iron, magnesium, zinc, copper, mercury, manganese and selenium. The highest death rates were found in mining areas (current or previous) having primary industries associated with greater levels of exposure to one or more of these metals.

Defective equipment and human error can aggravate this problem. Such was the case with poisoning of the Annapolis (Maryland) water supply from treatment with excessive fluoride (see below). If not monitored, hazardous amounts of mercury, lead, cadmium, chromium and manganese can leak into ground water from eroding landfills at municipal and private dumps.

I. Mercury

The threat of neurotoxicity from mercury continues to increase. Large outbreaks of mercury poisoning have occurred in the United States, Japan, Argentina and Iraq.

Sarafian and Verity (1993) demonstrated changes involving protein metabolism (phosphorylation) in cultured neurons after exposure to low concentrations of methyl mercury.

Mercury contamination has become a worldwide problem resulting from (1) the presence of this metal in numerous products (e.g., fungicides; electronic components; batteries), and (2) its release into the air and water from garbage incinerators, medical waste incinerators, coal- and oil-burning power plants, and some manufacturing operations. The contamination of fish illustrates the problem.

- Fish in the waterways of 26 states have been found to contain dangerously high levels of mercury.

- The fish in only 55 of 127 Florida waterways had sufficiently low levels of mercury to be considered acceptable for unlimited consumption (*The Miami Herald* January 24, 1993, p. B-1).

Daily intake. The estimated daily intake of mercury from air, water and food (exclusive of amalgam dental fillings) averages 3.0 micrograms (μg); 2.2 μg are absorbed (Lorscheider 1991). The upper daily limit of mercury suggested by the FDA is 2.89 μg. Humans absorb about 75 percent of the total daily intake of mercury from food.

Sources. Mercury contamination can result from diverse <u>industrial activities</u>. They include battery manufacture, mercury processing in drug and chemical factories, gold-mining operations, and oil exploration.

Many mercury-containing products—such as thermometers, batteries, paints, plastics, dyes, electronics, and fluorescent light bulbs—are discarded in <u>incinerators</u>, which then emit mercury into the environment.

- Mercury in fluorescent lamps escapes when the tubes are burned in incinerators, or crushed and buried in landfills. This has caused widespread contamination of ground water and lakes (*The Wall Street Journal* August 31, 1992, p. 8-2).

- The incineration of amalgam dental fillings (see below) during cremation exposes persons in many areas to mercury.

- Incinerators in South Florida's three large counties discharge an estimated 6,000 pounds mercury annually. This hazard is evidenced by the high mercury content in fish and raccoons, and the death of Florida panthers attributed to poisoning by mercury from eating contaminated fish (see above).

There are <u>other sources</u> of mercury exposure.

- The annual torching of more than 400,000 acres of sugar cane in the Everglades farm belt of South Florida, preparatory to harvesting and refining, releases an estimated 21,500 pounds mercury into the environment (Cook 1991).

- Mercury compounds were used as a mildew retardant in one-third of the 400 million gallons latex paint sold annually in the United States prior to 1990. High concentrations of mercury can persist in household air for months after interior walls are painted.

- Amalgam for dental fillings continues to be dumped illegally into water supplies.

The Issue of Dental Fillings. *The potential neurotoxicity of mercury in dental fillings has caused some dentists and physicians to recommend their removal, and* *replacement with other materials.* There have been reports of apparent dramatic remission of severely dementing illness following the removal of mercury fillings.

The limitations of laboratory testing were noted earlier. Blood mercury concentrations are an <u>unreliable</u> diagnostic index of chronic low-dose mercury exposure from dental amalgams. Tissue mercury levels can be high even though blood concentrations may be low.

Some governmental bodies have reacted to this danger.

- California initiated a "Dental Informed Consent Law" (SB 934) as a result of awareness of potential mercury poisoning from dental fillings.

- The Federal Health Agency in Germany now advises the use of amalgam fillings only for molars (*The Lancet* 1992; 339:419). It banned amalgam containing gamma-2 (a compound of mercury and tin) because of its instability and the risk of mercury release during the dental procedure.

The following data pertain to "silver" fillings (Lorscheider 1991, Null 1992).

- The American Dental Association estimates that dentists insert more than 100 million amalgam fillings annually in the United States.

- A single amalgam filling weighs 1.5-2.0 grams. Fifty percent is elemental mercury.

- Each surface of amalgam leaches at least one microgram (μg) mercury daily. Accordingly, a person with 10 fillings (each piece having three surfaces) potentially could be exposed to 30 μg mercury daily.

- The mercury absorbed by individuals with many amalgam fillings can be as high as 100 μg daily!

- The acts of prolonged brushing, grinding the teeth, chewing gum, and drinking hot fluid increase the rate of mercury vapor released from amalgam fillings (*The Lancet* 1992; 339:419).

<u>Mercury Accumulation in Brain Tissue</u>. A direct correlation has been reported between the number of dental amalgams and the amount of mercury present in brain (Null 1992). Persons with five or more amalgams averaged three times more mercury in the brain at autopsy than those with no amalgam.

Analysis of the brains of AD patients and age-matched control groups for trace elements revealed considerably more mercury in the former (Bjorklund 1991). Moreover, it tends to concentrate in the cerebral cortex and nucleus basalis of Meynert, the major cholinergic projection (Chapter 4).

II. <u>Lead</u>

Lead is neurotoxic, especially for children. Dr. Herbert L. Needleman (1992) reviewed human lead exposure and its neurobiological effects. The problem requires constant vigilance and careful control (see Chapter 17).

Although stronger regulatory restraints have been introduced, extensive and often unrecognized exposure to lead persists. Moreover, young children are affected by lead at far <u>lower levels</u> than formerly thought to be safe... often with many subtle adverse effects (see below).

There are multiple sources of lead exposure. They include lead solder in the seams of cans (mostly imported) containing food and beverages, lead-glazed ceramic dishware, leaded gasoline, lead-based paint and its dust, pesticides, and hair dyes used by men.

- FDA Commissioner David A. Kessler stated that 90 percent of all canned goods sold during 1979 were in lead-soldered containers (*The Miami Herald* June 22, 1993, p. C-1). The lead from such solders, used to seal the side seams, can bleed through and contaminate the contents.

- There has been a striking increase in sales of hair-coloring products used by men, especially "baby boomers" (*The Wall Street Journal* March 2, 1993, p. B-1).

- Some herbal medicines, such as hai ge fen (or clamshell powder), have resulted in lead poisoning (Markowitz 1994).

Testing. There are four chief methods for detecting or confirming the presence of excessive lead.

- <u>Measurement of whole blood lead by graphite-furnace, atomic absorption spectroscopy.</u> A concentration of 10 micrograms (μg) per 100 ml—0.5μmol per liter, or 100 parts per billion (ppb)—is the threshold of concern for the Centers for Disease Control (CDC). However, adverse effects on intelligence, hearing and growth, as well as transplacental lead transfer, can occur below this limit.

- <u>Measurement of lead in the hair by emission spectroscopy.</u> Levels greater than 5 parts per million (ppm) in children, or greater than 10 ppm in adults, are significant.

- <u>Analysis of lead in 24-hour urine specimens.</u> Concentrations exceeding 0.06 mg/24 hours in adults, or more than 0.04 ppm in a non-provoked urine specimen (i.e., without exposure to a lead chelating or complexing agent before the collection), are suspicious.

- <u>Measurement of zinc-complexed protoporphyrins in red blood cells</u>. Levels above 35 μg per 100 ml packed cells should suggest inhibition of protoporphyrin metabolism by a heavy metal such as lead.

Oral Intake. Lead-contaminated <u>drinking water</u> contributes up to 20 percent of the total lead exposure in young children.

The Environmental Protection Agency (EPA) disclosed that excessive levels of lead existed in the drinking water of 130 cities—including New York, Detroit, and Washington, D.C. (Gutfeld 1992). It also estimated that 32 million persons in the United States drink water from systems in which the lead content exceeds 15 parts per billion (ppb)… considered the upper "safe" limit. (The concentration exceeded 70 ppb in ten cities, with a high of 211 ppb in Charleston, South Carolina.)

More recently, the EPA reported that more than 10 percent of the United States population draws its drinking water from systems that contain unsafe levels of lead—i.e., more than 15 ppb (Noah 1993). Lead levels tended to be higher in small cities having less sophisticated treatment facilities. They included Grosse Pointe Park, Michigan (324 ppb); Goose Creek, South Carolina (257 ppb); and Honesdale, Pennsylvania (210 ppb). The extraordinary level of 484 ppb found at Camp Lajeune, a U.S. Marine Corps base in North Carolina, largely stemmed from lead-lined coolers in drinking fountains.

The striking increase of lead in drinking fluoridated water is discussed under fluoride (see below).

Lead also may be present contained in <u>unsuspected products.</u>

- High concentrations of lead (exceeding the statutory limit of 1 ppm) are present in some <u>imported ethnic foods</u>—e.g., Asian pickles; canned okra.

- The lead present in bronze and brass equipment can contaminate <u>draft beers</u>.

- <u>Wine</u> may contain considerable lead, especially expensive imported products. Levels ranging from 50 ppb to 700 ppb were found in ALL wines tested by the U.S. Bureau of Alcohol, Tobacco and Firearms, especially imports (Deveny 1991). The sources were tin-coated lead capsules used to cap wine bottles (now being phased out), the lead foil wrappers of wine bottles, old lead pipes in the vats at some wineries, and soil contamination.

Lead vapor. Inhaled lead vapor is neurotoxic. A pertinent epidemiologic study conducted by the Mayo Clinic involved 74 patients with amyotrophic lateral sclerosis (ALS) and 201 matched controls (Armon 1991). There was a higher incidence of ALS among men who worked at welding, soldering, and other blue-collar jobs than in the controls.

Vulnerability of Children. Neurotoxicity among children from lead exposure continues to be widespread. Levels of lead contracted in early childhood persist at least several years (Baghurst 1992). Furthermore, its ravages exist among all social and economic classes—that is, unattributable to factors such as poverty, lower social class, or an urban environment.

- Government statistics indicate that two million children live in housing containing old lead-based paint (Spears 1991).

- The U.S. Public Health Service estimates that up to four million children have blood lead levels sufficiently high (i.e., above 10-15 µg per 100 ml) to cause mental and behavioral problems (Spears 1991)!

Young children may be exposed to lead in various ways. They include infant formulas, the eating of chips or flakes of lead paint (particularly in pre-1970 housing), food in lead-soldered cans, soldered joints used in copper plumbing to carry drinking water, and exposure to the exhausts of metal smelters.

Shannon and Graef (1992) reported the hazard of infant formulas reconstituted with lead-contaminated water. The sources might be the first water drawn in the morning, and the prolonged boiling of water (especially in lead-containing kettles).

New guidelines by the Centers for Disease Control suggest intervention with blood levels of 10 µg per 100 ml (0.5 µmol per liter) or higher.

III. <u>Fluoride</u>

Fluoride neurotoxicity remains a controversial subject. It is addressed here because the population increasingly has been exposed to fluoride since the mid-1940s.

The following information is amplified in my solicited commentary (Roberts 1992c) for *Review of Fluoride: Benefits and Risks*, published in February 1991 by the Public Health Service.

- Fluoride is a toxic by-product of industry.

- Fluoride compounds (sodium fluoride; stannous fluoride; sodium monofluo-rophosphate) have <u>not</u> been shown to be essential for human metabolism.

- Community-wide fluoridated water is being consumed by <u>half</u> the United States population.

- The level of "optimal fluoridation" for drinking water has been established at one part per million (ppm).

- The recommended total daily intake of fluoride is 1 mg.

- A 1985 EPA study estimated that 13.8 million persons were exposed to fluoridated public drinking water containing in excess of 1-2 mg/L.

- Children and adults frequently ingest 4-5 times more than the recommended intake.

- Fluoride also is ingested in many products—e.g., toothpaste, mouth washes, therapeutic dental gels, vitamin-mineral supplements, infant formulas, and even sodas and food processed in municipalities where water is fluoridated.

- A survey of 153 pediatricians and 14 pediatric dentists in the Houston area revealed that 96 percent (!) of the participants prescribed fluoride supplements, generally until 16 years of age (Jones 1992).

Fluoride toxicity. Fluoride inhibits protein and DNA synthesis in mammalian cells. It therefore can cause chromosomal alterations, and alter or inhibit a wide variety of enzymes and enzymatic processes. Some of these processes involve important metabolic activities within the brain related to acetylcholine metabolism (Chapter 5) and the availability of glucose (Chapter 8). For example, up to 61 percent of acetylcholinesterase activity may be inhibited by the presence of 1 ppm fluoride (Froede 1985, Yiamouyiannis 1986).

> Gilbert's syndrome is a benign liver disorder in which the circulating unconjugated bilirubin concentration (characteristic of jaundice) is increased. One of the mechanisms probably involves inhibition of a liver enzyme (glucuronyl transferase) that conjugates bilirubin. Lee (1983) reported six patients with this disorder in whom increased plasma bilirubin decreased toward normal after switching from fluoridated to nonfluoridated water. (One patient was observed to have similar responses in three alternating periods of ingesting fluoridated and nonfluoridated water.)

Fluoridation has been championed by virtually every health professional as a 20th Century technological advance capable of preventing dental caries by itself. (This allegation has been challenged.) Unfortunately, such prophylaxis has potential systemic hazards.

- Small amounts of fluoride can have adverse effects on the immune system and on bone.

- At least three reports indicate increased fractures associated with chronic fluorosis (fluoride accumulation).

- There is evidence that excessive fluoride can have synergistic adverse effects both on the nervous and circulatory systems in persons exposed to other toxic elements, such as arsenic (Yue-Zhen 1992).

Fluoride and the Brain. The adverse effects of excessive fluoride on brain function make it suspect as a risk factor for AD.

Fluoride is rapidly and almost completely absorbed from the gastrointestinal tract. (Since it also enters the breast milk, young infants can be exposed to significant amounts.) Furthermore, the nervous system may be exposed chronically to fluoride because of its ready release from bone with aging and other conditions (e.g., acidosis). These facts are pertinent:

- Fluoride and aluminum added to drinking water cause behavioral changes in rats, and a loss of brain cells in the neocortex and hippocampus (Isaacson 1992).

- The brain content of fluoride increased from 0.53 ppm in 1939 (prior to water fluoridation) to 1.5 ppm in 1960-65 (Yiamouyiannis 1986). Although the blood-brain barrier (see above) is relatively impermeable to fluoride, it can be altered by certain influences, such as the action of aluminum (Chapter 10).

- Excessive fluoride was dumped into the Annapolis (Maryland) public water system on November 11, 1979. Some 10,000 persons developed acute fluoride poisoning; 65 percent of them complained of neurologic symptoms.

- Adverse brain effects may result from long-term fluoride exposure. They include headache, ringing in the ears, depression, confusion, drowsiness, visual disturbances, severe fatigue, and memory loss.

Fluoride and the Leaching of Lead. An incident in Tacoma (Washington) confirmed the ability of fluoride to leach lead from water pipes. The municipal water quality coordinator submitted an official report to the Department of Health indicating that the lead content rose nearly 100 percent during fluoridation, compared to the concentration when fluoridation was halted after the equipment broke down (*Chemical & Engineering News* December 13, 1993, p. 5). Specifically, the lead concentration was 17 ppb in the absence of fluoridation, and 32 ppb during fluoridation.

IV. Iron

The inclusion of iron as a neurotoxic element may surprise readers in view of the widespread promotion of numerous "enriched" or "fortified" foods (Chapter 7), and of vitamin-mineral "supplements" purported to maintain health and overcome "tired blood".

Iron Intake and Balance. The FDA suggests 18 mg iron as the recommended daily allowance (RDA)—the amount contained in a bowl of Kellogg's Product 19®.

The "optimal" daily allowance for iron ranges from 15-25 mg for men, and 20-30 mg for women. Since it is present in both animal products (meat, fish, poultry) and plant foods, there is generally no need to consume vitamin-mineral products containing iron.

There has been a tendency to overdiagnose "iron deficiency" in the absence of gross nutritional deficiency states and considerable blood loss through menstruation or gastrointestinal bleeding. Iron ingested in modest doses is clearly beneficial for women with iron-deficiency anemia caused by menstruation. With no other significant means for excreting iron, the body maintains iron balance chiefly by limiting its absorption (Crosby 1992).

- The intestinal lining has an extraordinarily efficient mechanism for absorbing only enough iron to offset small daily losses or to meet increased requirements associated with menstrual blood loss and pregnancy.

- Whenever this complicated system breaks down, the gut may absorb unneeded iron, which is conducive to overload.

Iron Toxicity. Excessive accumulation of iron can result from the consumption of "enriched" or "fortified" foods, and daily iron supplements. (Some regard the high content of iron in such products as "the snake oil of the 20th Century.") The ensuing increase of iron stores seems conducive to degenerative brain disease, metabolic dysfunction, and cardiac disorders—including heart attacks (Stripp 1992).

- Some believe that there is dysfunction of transferrin, the protein transporting iron, in persons with AD.

- Iron is deposited in the brain in AD and Parkinson's disease (Chapter 15).

- Sengstock, Alanow and Arendash (1993) induced progressive reduction in striatal dopamine in rats with a single infusion of low-dose iron into the substantia nigra, the area most affected in Parkinson's disease. This was accompanied by progressive biochemical and behavioral changes.

- Elevated iron stores may induce insulin antagonism (Pozza 1968) (Chapter 8). Conversely, the administration of desferrioxamine, a specific chelator of iron, has effected better control of diabetes (Cutler 1989).

- The ingestion of iron can interfere with thyroid metabolism. Campbell et al (1992) demonstrated that the simultaneous ingestion of ferrous sulfate and thyroxine reduces thyroxine efficiency, probably by binding iron to thyroxine.

The U.S. Preventive Services Task Force (1993) has asserted that there is little evidence routine iron supplementation during pregnancy benefits the clinical outcome for the mother, the fetus or the newborn. The adverse effects may include serious gastrointestinal complaints, birth defects, heart disease, infection, metabolic imbalances of other minerals, and potentially harmful elevated hemoglobin levels.

Excess iron in tissues can become a "metabolic loose cannon." The "free radicals" so generated are capable of causing injury through various mechanisms, including damage to DNA, enzymes, and the integrity of cell membranes (Stripp 1992). Free iron tends to promote formation of the highly toxic hydroxyl radical involved in lipid peroxidation. Moreover, aluminum (Chapter 10) interacts with iron and its carrier transferrin.

The role of iron in diseases related to oxidant injury is illustrated by the retinopathy of prematurity and bronchopulmonary dysplasia. Premature infants are more susceptible to the adverse effects of excess iron due to immaturity of their antioxidant mechanisms (Chang-Enger 1993).

V. <u>Arsenic</u>

Recurrent nonhomicidal exposure to arsenic in food, water and air can result in neurotoxicity, especially as the pentavalent salt. It is evidenced by altered function of the brain and peripheral nerves (polyneuropathy), and liver, thyroid, kidney and bone marrow changes.

The sources of arsenic are multiple. They include the following:

- Polluted air from the smelting of copper, lead, zinc and other ores, the burning of coal, glass makers, and other plants that emit arsenic (also causing skin and lung cancer)

- Industrial use as an additive to metal alloys, wood preservatives, and the production of glass, paints and textiles

- Sprays and other products used as pesticides and rodenticides that contain arsenic

- Well water contaminated by toxic dumps, and by nearby asbestos or other plants

- The leaching of arsenic into hot springs from rocks and soil (reported in the United States, Taiwan, Japan and New Zealand)

- The use of arsenicals and arsanilic acid as feed additives for poultry and live-stock

- Batches of dolomite and bonemeal taken as calcium supplements (Roberts 1981a,b; 1983a)

- Arsenical ores used in some areas as seasoning in place of onion or garlic

The frequency and amounts of arsenic in various foods are noteworthy (Millichap 1993). They include meat, shellfish, poultry and cow's milk. Concentrations up to 1,500 ppb in milk have resulted from cows grazing in arsenic-contaminated fields.

Batches of bottled water contaminated with arsenic also have been found. Three of 28 brands of sparkling water were identified by *Consumer Reports* in January 1987 as containing concentrations exceeding the federal standards.

DRUG NEUROTOXICITY

The widespread availability of potent drugs that can profoundly affect brain function represents another 20th Century phenomenon. Their use must be considered a risk factor for AD, especially with aging.

- A 1989 report submitted to the House Select Committee on Aging by Inspector General Richard Kusserow (U.S. Health and Human Services Department) indicated that the average older person annually takes more than 15 prescriptions.

- Overmedication of the elderly is illustrated by the estimate of Dr. Peter Lamy (University of Maryland School of Pharmacy) that 10 to 20 percent of all emergency room admissions of elderly patients result from overmedication (*The Palm Beach Post* March 24, 1993, p. D-5). He warned older persons: "Don't ascribe anything to aging, particularly if you're prescribed a new drug or new dosage."

Potentially, many drugs can damage nerve cells and interfere with neurotransmitters. They include prescription, over-the-counter, and illicit products.

Other factors may compound this situation, such as the lessened ability to handle drugs due to liver and kidney disease, and with aging. Experimental evidence has shown alterations in the blood-brain barrier from age-related changes in microvessels of the hippocampus—but not in other cerebral cortical areas or its white matter (Mooradian 1993).

There is increased awareness of adverse effects from relatively small dosages of standard drugs, even in normal subjects. For example, Caplan et al (1993) noted that doses of oral theophylline, a drug often employed in treating asthma, can cause significant disturbances in sleep quality among normal persons. It reduced total sleep time by approximately one-half hour, and increased the number of arousals by four episodes per hour.

The striking effects of some drugs on other species are sobering. For example, allopurinol (a drug used to relieve gout by preventing the accumulation of uric acid crystals in joints) renders female cockroaches unable to reproduce—and thus could decimate an entire population of this species.

The risk-versus-benefit aspect of drug therapy also must be considered. For example, it is unlikely that a few conventional doses of antihistamine drugs, such as diphenhydramine (Benadryl®), will induce attention deficits comparable to that of AD patients in the absence of underlying pathology.

I. Psychotropic Drugs

Various popular "nerve medicines" alter or deplete important neurotransmitters—most notably serotonin, dopamine, and norepinephrine (Chapter 5). For example, the antidepressant fluoxetine hydrochlorida (Prozac®) inhibits serotonin uptake by the brain, and enhances the action of norepinephrine.

Clinical problems associated with the use of triazolam (Halcion®) illustrate such concern. Its administration at bedtime can result in memory impairment and amnesia the following day (Bixler 1991). These effects do not appear to occur with temazepam (Restoril®). Significant changes in delayed recall also may develop after taking triazolam.

The extent of such drug usage is extraordinary.

- One-third of persons who use daily benzodiazepines in the United States are 55 years or older. Examples of these drugs are Librium® and Valium®. They have been referred to as "the only routinely prescribed addicting drugs."

- Up to three percent of individuals in the Western world have received benzodiazepine therapy continuously for more than one year. Such consumption has been greater among women and older persons.

The cumulative adverse effects of long-acting benzodiazepines in the elderly reflect their prolonged metabolism—that is, over weeks. Neuropsychologic testing has confirmed the prolonged impairment of learning and memory in older patients after benzodiazepine detoxification (Rummaus 1993), even when no outward signs of withdrawal were evident. This included impaired ability to learn new information (anterograde amnesia).

II. General Anesthetics

The possible contributory role of general anesthetic drugs to AD requires reevaluation. At low concentrations, these agents inhibit the respiration of brain tissue (Elliott 1962), and reduce brain cell activity (Brunner 1971).

The short-term use of anesthetics can impair car driver performance (Poldinger 1968).

Occupational exposure to high levels of nitrous oxide, used in dental offices for anesthesia, has been linked to systemic problems. They include psychomotor deficits, sperm abnormalities, birth defects, spontaneous abortion, and reduced fertility (Rowland 1992).

The prolonged hypoxemia after general anesthesia will be discussed in Chapter 12.

106

III. Appetite-Suppressing Drugs

Many individuals with a problem of overweight, real or perceived, resort to pharmacologic measures. The use of appetite-suppressing drugs (so-called "diet pills") for weight loss could have long-term consequences involving brain function, especially in conjunction with low-calorie products that contain aspartame (Chapter 9). Such prescription pills include fenfluramine (Pondimin®) and phentimine (Ionamin®; Adipex-P®; Fastin®; Phentermine HCL®).

More pointedly, weight-conscious women who turn to these measures risk malnutrition, severe hypoglycemia (Chapter 7) and brain damage through the combination of excessive caloric restriction, the prodigious consumption of aspartame-sweetened "diet" drinks, and neurotoxic appetite-suppressing drugs.

Fenfluramine has been prescribed as an appetite suppressant for two decades. It belongs to a class of amphetamine-related drugs that includes methylphenidate (Ritalin®) (generally not toxic, even at high doses), and the illegal drug "ecstasy" (3,4-methylene-dioxymethamphetamine; MDMA).

Fenfluramine is a 50-50 combination of dexfenfluramine and levofenfluramine. Fenfluramine—especially its dexfenfluramine component—selectively damages the fine nerve endings (terminals) of brain cells that release serotonin (Barnes 1989), and decreases overall brain levels of this neurotransmitter. It can also kill groups of nerve cells. Its administration for only four days to squirrels can cause extensive brain damage still detectable 1-1/2 years later.

IV. Drugs of Abuse

All drugs of abuse are potentially neurotoxic. Some examples:

- Phencyclidine (PCP) (Olney 1989)
- 1-methyl-4-phenyl-1,2,3,6 tetrahydrophyridine (MPTP), a synthetic heroin that selectively destroys dopamine-containing nerve cells
- Certain amphetamine analogues that can damage central "monoaminergic neurons"—i.e., dopamine neurons by amphetamine; serotonin neurons by MDMA; and both types by methamphetamine

AIR POLLUTION: CARBON MONOXIDE POISONING

General Considerations

Air pollution has become an enormous problem of global proportions. Cities, national parks and whole countries are encountering diminished air quality. Contributory factors include scores of environmental pollutants, acid rain, depletion of the ozone layer, and the "greenhouse effect."

The problem of polluted indoor air has been compounded by inadequate flow rates of fresh air in many "energy efficient" homes and commercial buildings. The "sick building syndrome" is being encountered more frequently.

The following data provide a partial overview (Krupnick (1991):

- More than 66 million Americans live in counties where the ozone standard was exceeded at one or more monitors during 1989.

- Another 27.4 million persons live in areas where the particulate standards for air have been violated—viz., 0.1 part per million (ppm) for sulfur dioxide; 8.5 ppm for nitrogen dioxide; 33.6 ppm for carbon monoxide.

The role of carbon monoxide and other environmental neurotoxins as potential risk factors for AD are discussed below.

Carbon Monoxide Exposure

Nonlethal carbon monoxide poisoning represents an epidemic that is not fully appreciated. An estimated 10,000 persons in the United States seek medical attention or miss work annually because of exposure to carbon monoxide.

This colorless and non-irritating gas is generated by incomplete combustion in machine engines. The initial effects of carbon monoxide inhalation include lowered attention, difficult concentration, sleepiness, mental lethargy, and muscular incoordination. These symptoms have been clearly documented in drivers (McFarland 1962).

Carbon monoxide reaches the highest concentration of any gaseous pollutant in the urban atmosphere (Roberts 1971b). *Accordingly, it deserves consideration as a risk factor for the development of AD.*

Frequent Sources. Carbon monoxide can be inhaled from the following sources:

- Smoking (Chapter 16)

- Motor vehicle exhausts (leaks due to faulty design or manufacturer error; emissions from surrounding vehicles) (Chapter 17)

- Vulnerable occupations (traffic policemen; highway tollbooth workers)

- Pedestrians (in areas of heavy traffic)

- Industrial waste

- Wood-burning stoves

- Defective water heaters, furnaces, and space heaters

- Improperly used or maintained gas lamps, ovens, and stoves in poorly-ventilated recreational vehicles

- Indoor industrial machinery

- Gasoline-powered resurfacing equipment in inadequately ventilated indoor ice-skating rinks (coupled with heaters used to heat the stands)

- Burning polyvinyl chloride (PVC) (widely used in carpets, furniture, wall coverings, and electrical insulation during the late 1960s)

The reports by Hampson et al (1993, 1994) of unintentional carbon monoxide poisoning in scores of patients following a winter storm that struck western Washington State on January 20, 1993 illustrate this ever-potential threat. The interruption of electrical power for an estimated 700,000 residents was coupled with near-freezing temperatures during the four nights following this storm. Exposure to carbon monoxide increased as they resorted to alternative sources of energy for indoor cooking and home heating—especially gasoline-powered generators, propane-powered heaters in poorly ventilated areas, and the burning of charcoal briquettes.

Adverse Effects of Carbon Monoxide. Goldsmith and Landaw (1968) and others have reviewed the effects of carbon monoxide on human health. Most involve hypoxemia (Chapter 12) because it interferes with oxygen transport.

Human hemoglobin has a far greater affinity for carbon monoxide than for oxygen. The resulting formation of carboxyhemoglobin decreases the release of oxygen carried by hemoglobin.

Carbon monoxide exposure can cause brain changes. Such poisoning has resulted in "secondary" parkinsonism. Non-smoking adults who suffered acute carbon monoxide intoxication develop varying degrees of verbal and nonverbal memory impairment, even after prompt emergency hyperbaric treatment (Fennell 1991).

OTHER ENVIRONMENTAL NEUROTOXINS

A congressional hearing on *Neurotoxins: At Home And The Workplace* (see above), *conducted in 1986 by the Committee on Science and Technology, concluded that exposure to neurotoxins is one of the top ten causes of illness and injury in the United States workforce.* The National Research Council (1992) underscored the need for vigorously pursuing reports of neurotoxicity in *Environmental Neurotoxicology.*

The EPA reported that the chemical industry produced about half of the 5.7 billion pounds of toxins annually generated nationwide (McMurray 1991). The toxins include solvents, benzene, herbicides and insecticides. Regulatory standards existed or had been recommended for only 167 of the 850 known neurotoxic chemicals covered. Moreover, few tests specifically directed to neurotoxicity were being conducted.

Recognition of the mounting importance of neurotoxins and their relation to neurodegeneration, notably Parkinson's disease, is reflected at various symposia (e.g., New York Academy of Sciences, 1992) and hearings held by regulatory agencies. Neurotoxins causing prolonged imbalance of brain neurotransmitters could "result in devastating neurological or psychiatric disorders that impair the quality of life, cripple and potentially reduce the highest intellect to a vegetative state" (*loc. cit.*, U.S. Government Printing Office, 1989). Unborn and young children, who lack the fully developed toxicologic defense mechanisms of adults, are uniquely vulnerable to such exposure.

A few selected classes of environmental neurotoxins will be reviewed, followed by a discussion of the controversial but pertinent subject of multiple chemical sensitivity (MCS).

I. Pesticides and Herbicides

The use of organophosphate insecticides that affect acetylcholinesterase, the enzyme acting on acetylcholine (Chapter 5), rose dramatically after the mid-century. Herbicides are now among the highest-volume chemicals.

The EPA estimated that at least 25 million pounds of herbicides and 30 million pounds of insecticides were applied annually to residential lawns and gardens over the past decade—often by inadequately trained persons who did not take necessary precautions to safeguard against inhalation. For aesthetic reasons only, homeowners used nearly six times more pesticide per acre than farmers (Skow 1991)!

The Environmental Working Group reported the extraordinary degree of pesticide residues in various fruits and vegetables, based on 1990-1992 data compiled by the Environmental Protection Agency (*The New York Times* June 27, 1993, p. 11). Residues were found in 59 percent of 4,468 samples tested! The percentages were as follows: strawberries 82%; cherries 80%; oranges 80%; peaches 79%; apples 68%; celery 75%; pears 73%; lettuce 68%; spinach 54%; carrots 50%. This group also stated that millions of children in the United States have received up to 35 percent of their entire lifetime dose of some carcinogenic pesticides by the age of five.

The neurotoxicity of pesticide residues has been convincingly shown in animal studies (Millichap 1993). Minute amounts can cause impairment of learning and memory, hyperactivity, and aggressive behavior.

I have received detailed letters from observant persons who, along with members of their family, experienced memory problems ("real blank times"), constant headaches, debilitating fatigue and other symptoms following the direct or indirect exposure to "cide" chemicals. This entailed spraying of their houses, walking on treated golf courses, and consuming coffee or other products so treated.

The neurotoxicity of these chemicals has been repeatedly documented. Children are highly vulnerable to pesticide mists.

- Even a single episode of organophosphate poisoning might result in chronic neurophysiologic dysfunction (Rosenstock 1991).

- The neurotoxicity of occupationally-used herbicides extends to Parkinson's disease (Semchuk 1992).

- Drugs such as cimetidine (Tagamet®) can enhance the toxicity of pesticides (Allen 1991).

II. Neurotoxicity From Other Chemical Exposures

Neurologic injury can be sustained both by workers and consumers who are exposed to a variety of chemicals. It is especially likely after prolonged low-level exposure to those substances having long-term effects. The fetus is highly vulnerable.

Xintaras et al (1979) noted that adverse effects of neurotoxins tend to become clinically evident with age and after repeated exposure to chemical stress. Earlier detection might be possible by means of a battery of performance tests that measure cognition, perception and psychomotor abilities.

This issue is illustrated by exposure to toluene (methyl benzene). It is a component of spray paints, glues, lacquers, adhesives and cleaning liquids. These products are used widely in woodworking and dry cleaning industries, industrial chemical operations, and the environment of artists. Chronic inhalation of this solvent can result in cognitive impairment, tremor, severe unsteadiness (ataxia), and diffuse atrophy of the brain (Rosenberg 1991).

Even the inhalation of gasoline vapors by motorists who pump at self-service stations must be regarded with suspicion for neurotoxicity.

III. Multiple Chemical Sensitivity (MCS)

The frequency and severity of neurobehavioral changes resulting from exposure to many environmental chemicals continue to be debated. Based on its 18-month study, the

National Academy of Sciences suggested that *15 percent of the population may experience "increased allergic sensitivity" to chemicals* (National Research Council 1987). The offending chemicals exist in many common household products —e.g., detergents, solvents, pesticides, metals and rubber.

The dramatic rise of this problem during recent decades coincides with the escalating epidemicity of AD.

> Using single-photon emission computed tomography (SPECT) scanning, Callender (1991) reported that 56 of 67 patients with well-defined chemical exposures evidenced decreased flow in the frontal and temporal lobes, and in the basal ganglia. Similar results were found in several patients by PET scanning—i.e., reduced brain glucose metabolism involving the hippocampus, amygdala, putamen and thalamus. *Comparable findings exist in "early" AD* (Chapters 4 and 5).

Different names have been used to describe the clinical syndromes resulting from chemical-induced sensitivity. They are "multiple chemical sensitivity syndrome" (MCS), "universal allergy," "the total allergy syndrome," "environmental allergy," "cerebral allergy," the environmental maladaption syndrome," and "20th Century disease." Clinical ecologists, however, stress that the MCS syndrome is not associated with altered immunoglobulins, as with conventional "allergies."

Dr. H. Hugh Fudenberg (1993), an investigator of immune dysfunction in AD (Chapter 6), estimated that one-half (!) of patients diagnosed as AD in a South Carolina state hospital had *treatable* chemical hypersensitivity… especially to petrochemicals.

The MCS Syndrome. Dr. Theron Randolph (1980, 1987), a pioneer in this field, described the severe effects of noxious environmental agents on susceptible individuals. They include headache (the most common symptom), hyperactivity, dizziness, anxiety attacks, severe depression, impaired thinking ("brain fag"), memory loss, flu-like symptoms, extreme fatigue, and gastrointestinal complaints (especially among children).

The exposure of these persons even to trace amounts of chemicals in common foods or indoor air can induce or reproduce symptoms, especially the "sick building syndrome" (see below). The offending substances might be petrochemicals, MSG (Chapter 9), sulfites, formaldehyde, pesticide residues, paint fumes, deodorants, scented detergents, colored ink in magazines, artificial colors, sweeteners (Chapter 9), preservatives, ripening procedures (e.g., ethylene gas), protective food waxes, plastics food wraps, other packaging materials, the phenolic resin found in some can linings, and butylated compounds used with rubber gaskets to seal food containers.

- Carpeting and adhesives can emit toxic chemicals indoors. Furthermore, carpeting may act as a "sink" for pesticides, molds and dust mites. As many as 120 chemicals have been identified in carpeting and the carpeting underlayments used for installation. Many are known to be toxic and carcinogenic —e.g., benzene, toluene, xylene, styrene, and solvent-based dyes.

- The "sick building syndrome" can result from many sources. In addition to carpeting and poorly maintained heating and cooling systems, they include carbonless paper (alkylphenol novalac resin), photocopiers (phthalates; isocyanates; xylene), laser printers (styrene-butadiene), computer terminals, dry-process copiers (ozone), dry-cleaned fabrics (perchloroethylene), and partitions/paneling (formaldehyde; benzene; methylene chloride; perchloroethylene; xylene).

Vulnerable Groups. Ashford and Miller (1989) listed these four groups or clusters of persons who are highly sensitive to low-level chemical exposure:

- Industrial workers with acute and chronic exposure to industrial chemicals
- Occupants of "tight buildings" exposed to tobacco smoke, inadequate ventilation, and construction materials and furnishings in new buildings
- Residents of communities that are subjected to considerable chemical contamination from toxic waste sites, aerial pesticide spraying, ground water contamination, and air contamination from industry
- Persons who evidence reactions to chemicals such as pesticides, drugs and consumer products

12

THE ROLE OF DECREASED BRAIN OXYGEN

It is the theory which decides what we can observe.

Albert Einstein

... there is good evidence of reduced cerebral oxygen uptake in dementia, and reduced acetylcholine synthesis occurs when glucose oxidation is impaired by mild hypoxia.

D. M. Bowen et al (1979)

Recurrent and prolonged decrease of oxygen to the brain (cerebral hypoxia or hypoxemia) can contribute to Alzheimer's disease (AD) because the brain is absolutely dependent upon a continuous and adequate oxygen supply. Accordingly, any influences that significantly lower the blood oxygen concentration and its delivery to the brain are likely to injure nerve cells, especially in conjunction with the effects of neurotoxins described earlier.

The consequences of severe and sustained hypoxemia on brain function relative to cognitive impairment have been shown in healthy volunteers (Hornbein 1989). Moreover, cells in the hippocampus (Chapter 4), an area crucial to memory, appear uniquely vulnerable to decreased oxygen supply.

There are potential prophylactic and therapeutic implications. For example, anecdotal accounts of striking improved mentation and brain uptake with imaging studies following hyperbaric oxygen have been reported by several physicians (personal communications).

113

CONDITIONS CONDUCIVE TO CEREBRAL HYPOXIA

A number of conditions that decrease brain oxygenation constitute potential risk factors for AD. Most can be avoided or minimized through behavior modification (e.g., cessation of smoking), precautionary measures (e.g., the administration of oxygen postoperatively), and the adequate medical treatment of heart and lung diseases.

Smoking (Chapter 16)

This habit can result in hypoxemia—both directly through decreased oxygen uptake by the lungs, and indirectly from the effects of carbon monoxide (Chapter 11) (see below). Its adverse effects also are inflicted on innocent nonsmokers exposed to "passive smoke" or "sidestream smoke." The children of parents who smoke are highly vulnerable (Young 1991).

Prolonged Sleep

Excessive sleep from any cause may result in hypoxemia due to decreased ventilation. Also, it carries a risk of reduced glucose availability to the brain in persons prone to hypoglycemia who go four or more hours without nourishment (Chapter 8).

> Emphasizing the value of being an "early riser" to prevent premature aging, Lorand (1910, pp. 132 and 381) astutely noted: "Too much sleep may be nearly as bad as too little."

Excessive sleep can have other serious consequences. In a prospective epidemiologic study involving more than one million men and women monitored for six years, Hammond (1968) reported higher death rates at all ages among persons who usually slept nine or more hours at night.

Narcolepsy (Chapter 15)

Narcolepsy also requires attention. This common condition refers to excessive and inappropriate sleep. It is often misdiagnosed as other conditions, especially "chronic fatigue" (Chapter 16). I have stressed the frequent clinical association of narcolepsy and hypoglycemia (Roberts 1964, 1967b, 1971).

Sleep Apnea

Sleep apnea has been recognized increasingly as a major threat to health. This condition describes prolonged periods of nonbreathing during sleep, often terminated by severe snoring. Low blood oxygen concentrations occur during the extended periods of nonbreathing.

The significant cognitive impairment that may develop in patients with this disorder can improve dramatically with appropriate treatment (Scheltens 1991b). Therapy includes weight reduction, the avoidance of alcohol, smoking and sedatives, mechanical or surgical procedures that insure an adequate airway, and some drugs.

The Postoperative State

The marked degree of hypoxemia that occurs postoperatively (*The Lancet* 1992; 340:580-582) is not generally appreciated. Significant oxygen desaturation (below 85 percent) can persist for many hours to five days (!) after anesthesia. *Routine* postoperative oxygenation therefore should be considered, especially in patients having other AD risk factors.

Dental Anesthesia

The risk of hypoxemia during dental anesthesia has led to recommending stringent standards for dentists. They include certification in Advanced Cardiac Life Support (ACLS), and the training of staff members to monitor patients during "deep sedation" and "general anesthesia"—as with pulse oximetry (using a device that measures the blood oxygen content through the skin) (Rosenthal 1993).

Heart and Lung Disorders

Hypoxemia is a hallmark of heart failure, emphysema, and other lung conditions. Patients with these disorders often experience confusion at low oxygen concentrations, especially during the night.

Air Travel

Air travel is clearly a 20th Century phenomenon. Flying introduces the risk of hypoxemia, especially for persons who have the aforementioned medical disorders (Dillard 1991).

Commercial planes operate most efficiently at altitudes of 25,000-40,000 feet. However, their cabin pressures heretofore were pressurized (supercharged) at the equivalency of about 8,000-9,000 feet. Half of B-767 flights were found to have cabin conditions equivalent to 7412 feet or more above sea level (Cottrell 1988).

Exposure to carbon monoxide from inhaled smoking (see above) compounds the problem for passengers seated in nonsmoking areas when it is permitted during long flights.

"Stale air" in the cabins of new larger aircraft (including Boeing 757s and 767s, and McDonnell Douglas MD80s) could pose a related serious problem. In an era of fierce competition in which the use of less fuel to cool the outside air is emphasized, these newer models may provide half fresh air-half recirculated air that is freshened only every six to 12 minutes (Tolchin 1993). (This contrasts with 100 percent fresh air circulating every three minutes in aircraft built before the mid-1980s.) As a result, carbon monoxide and carbon dioxide levels tend to be higher, along with increased concentrations of cleaning agents, pesticides and benzene. Headaches, lightheadedness, dizziness and nausea have been attributed to such exposure, especially after long flights.

Other phenomena than reduced oxygen justify the "fear of flying." They include dehydration, spraying with pesticides (e.g., on international passengers disembarking in New Zealand), exposure to pesticides from treated cargo, exposure to formaldehyde and other toxic chemicals in cabin furnishings, and exposure to toxic chemicals from fuel exhaust (especially before takeoff).

- There is greater exposure to ozone above 35,000 feet, along with increased radiation exposure (Fairechild 1993).

- The risk of exposure to bacteria and viruses is increased in the economy section of larger planes (such as the 747). Pilots routinely turn off one-third of airflow to this area—but not to their own (Fairechild 1993).

High Altitude

Prolonged or recurrent exposure to high-altitude areas (e.g., mountainous communities; ski lodges and other facilities) places some individuals at risk of hypoxemia, especially without gradual acclimatization. The threshold for altitude-related illness is generally 8,000 feet (2,440 meters). At that level, the arterial oxygen pressure is 60 mm mercury, and the arterial oxygen saturation only 92 percent. Both decrease steeply at higher altitudes.

There has been increased awareness of the frequency of <u>acute mountain sickness</u> in a general population of visitors to moderate elevation, such as at 6300-9700 feet in the Rocky Mountains of Colorado.

- Honigman et al (1993) studied a cohort of 4212 adults over a 3-year period who attended conferences at resorts in this area. They found evidence of acute mountain sickness in 25 percent, especially among younger persons who lived at sea level, and the less physically fit. This disorder occurred in 65 percent of travelers within the first 12 hours of arrival, especially if there had been no prior acclimatization at lower levels. Headache was the most common symptom.

- Zaccaria et al (1993) demonstrated an increase of sympathetic activity during high altitude hypoxia in humans. It was evidenced by increased norepinephrine excretion, heart rate variability, and a significant decrease in the number and affinity of alpha-2 adrenergic receptors. Such down-regulation of platelet alpha-2 adrenergic receptor induced by sympathetic activation is part of the adaptive response to high altitude hypoxia.

<u>Chronic exposure to high altitudes</u> has added clinical significance in the present context. The frequency of migraine experienced at high altitude (see below and Chapter 15) illustrates the issue. A prevalence rate of 12.4 percent was found in a Peru mining town located 14,200 feet above sea level, but only in 3.5 percent of populations living at sea level (Arregui 1991).

Migraine

The spasm of cerebral blood vessels associated with migraine risks a reduction of oxygen (and glucose) to the brain, often evidenced clinically as gross neurologic deficits during attacks. Furthermore, the induced release of neurotoxic excitatory amino acids (see Chapter 9 and below) can initiate a vicious cycle. The increased glutamate concentrations in migraine sufferers (Ferrari 1990) is germane.

Hypoglycemia

Reduced oxygenation of brain cells is compounded by the "metabolic hypoxia" of low glucose concentrations during hypoglycemia. This subject was discussed in Chapter 8.

Diabetes Mellitus

Elevated blood glucose levels in poorly controlled diabetics cause metabolic changes within cells involving energy (referred to as impaired oxidation of NADH to NAD+). Since they mimic the effects of hypoxia on neural function, this phenomenon has been designated "hyperglycemic pseudohypoxia" (Williamson 1993).

Carbon Monoxide Poisoning

Repeated non-lethal exposure to carbon monoxide, with impaired tissue oxygenation, represents an occult epidemic that is not generally recognized (Chapters 8 and 11). Annually, an estimated 10,000 persons in the United States seek medical attention for this disorder or miss work because of it.

Hypoxia During Pregnancy

There is experimental evidence that maternal hypoxemia results in intrauterine growth retardation, perhaps through insulin-like growth factors and their binding proteins (Tapanainen 1993).

MECHANISMS OF BRAIN INJURY FROM REDUCED OXYGEN

Several major derangements of physiology occur when the brain is deprived of adequate oxygen. The interested reader can find detailed explanations of the following mechanisms in medical texts. Although technical, interested readers may wish some of the details... especially as they relate to the neurotoxic disturbances discussed in previous chapters.

Impaired Oxidative Phosphorylation

This phenomenon refers to decreased availability of energy within the brain and other tissues. Oxygen depletion interferes with the production of adenosine triphosphate (ATP), the transport of neurotransmitters across cell membranes, and protein synthesis.

Entry Of Excess Calcium Into Cells (Chapter 8)

Reduced ATP interferes with intricate control mechanisms for calcium entry, and the distribution of calcium within cells. Such changes activate enzymes (lipases; proteases; endonucleases) that can destroy neurons. It is of interest that tangle-bearing neurons (Chapter 4) found in autopsied AD patients contain increased amounts of calcium (Garruto 1984).

Glutamate-Aspartate Neurotoxicity (Chapters 9 and 11)

Potent endogenous neurotoxins are released when the oxygen concentration is low. The ensuing increased amounts of glutamate and aspartate emanating from cells play a significant role in brain injury (Tendler 1991).

- It is estimated that exposure to only one percent of the brain's glutamate content for five minutes can cause the death of brain cells (Choi 1991).

- Glutamate neurotoxicity activates calcium-sensitive proteases (see above).

Acetylcholine Derangements

Both the synthesis and release of acetylcholine within the central nervous system (Chapter 5) are restrained by normal oxygen and glucose concentrations. These processes become markedly stimulated at low levels, even to the point of causing convulsions (Feldberg 1945). Such repeated stress probably contributes to the "high output failure" of acetylcholine synthesis found in AD, along with the selective loss of strategic cholinergic neurons.

Decreased circulation to the brain (ischemia) can initiate comparable events.

Kumagae and Matsui (1991) found dramatic changes in the cholinergic system of rat brain during an ischemic episode and for 60 minutes thereafter. Following an initial increase of extracellular acetylcholine in the ischemic period, its concentration declined markedly with restoration of the blood supply. Acetylcholine synthesis from glucose in hippocampal cells remained low for two days after reperfusion.

Local Tissue Changes That Favor Alzheimer Plaque Formation

The stimulation of amyloid protein precursor (APP) (Chapter 4), with subsequent deposition of beta-amyloid, appears to be a widespread biological response by many tissues to injury, including hypoxemia (Regland 1992). Furthermore, the reduced pH (acidity) caused by oxygen lack may accelerate amyloid plaque formation, and prevent the breakdown (proteolysis) of beta-peptide (Barrow 1991).

The Free Radical Theory

There is considerable interest in the role of so-called free radicals relative to de generation of the nervous system, the cardiovascular system, and other organs. One popular theory avers that a highly reactive unstable oxygen molecule damages cell walls, chromosomes, DNA, and lipoprotein metabolism—with the generation of "bad" low-density-lipoprotein (LDL) cholesterol.

I have reviewed this theory and its shortcomings, especially as it pertains to the alleged value of various antioxidants for "rustproofing" the body as "free radicals scavengers" (Roberts 1993). These include vitamins A, C and E, selenium, zinc, and other substances. (Vitamins C and E also may function as prooxidants.) However, there are potential hazards from taking excessive amounts of vitamins A and E (Roberts 1981c, 1993).

Altered Insulin Secretion

Experimental studies confirm that hypoxia leads to inhibition of insulin secretion as a result of adrenal and sympathetic nervous system stimulation (Jackson 1993). This phenomenon could account for the decreased birth weight of infants born to mothers with severe diabetes… reflecting a reduction of growth-promoting effects of insulin and other metabolic changes (see above).

13

THE ROLE OF EMOTIONAL STRESS

Man does not die; he kills himself.

Seneca

*There is a sickness which puts some of us in distemper,
but I cannot name the disease; and it is
caught of you that yet are well.*

Shakespeare
(*The Winter's Tale* Act 1, Scene 2)

Immature and untutored responses to stress and prolonged emotional turmoil incurred by disappointment, misfortune and conflicts at home or work, and by societal upheavals probably contribute significantly to Alzheimer's disease (AD). There is evidence that stress can act as a trigger for "cellular suicide" in neurodegenerative diseases (Shaffer 1993).

The effects of stress tend to be particularly pernicious during the several decades wherein AD evolves (Chapter 6).

- There is increasing focus on <u>stress in childhood</u> as a result of urban and class-room congestion, crime, poverty, air and water pollution, and commuting conditions. The "Children's Stress Index" (created by Zero Population Growth) listed Houston, Los Angeles, Miami, El Paso and Fresno as the worst metropolitan areas in the United States (*The Miami Herald* May 26, 1993, p. A-1).

    The basis for severe anxiety in childhood may be more subtle. For example, the first children of affluent and permissive families often experience intense free-floating anxiety resulting from compulsive perfectionism and unrealistic expectations. The tragic results are evidenced even among "successful" adults after the age of 30 as the so-called Peter Pan Syndrome (Kiley 1983)—especially depression, loneliness, and family crises.

- <u>Working women</u> often are beset with considerable stress as they attempt to juggle job and family pressures. This is more likely for single mothers who work long hours, and also bear the responsibility for supporting or monitoring elderly parents. The adverse effects may be reflected by increased absenteeism and decreased productivity.

- <u>Other forms of stress</u> continually emerge, such as the impact of job layoffs and corporate cutbacks ("downsizing"), and living with fear or frustration (see below).

This chapter serves as an introduction to Chapter 19, which offers general advice about coping constructively with stress in contemporary society. Dr. Hans Selye aptly defined stress as "the rate of wear and tear on the body." Experimentally, its effects are evidenced as accelerated atherosclerosis, cataracts and other degenerative changes.

Psychoneuroimmunology

The following perspectives are consistent with the thrust of psychoneuroimmunology and neuroendocrinimmunology, an emerging discipline dealing with physical and psychological interactions (Reichlin 1993). Using sophisticated methods (e.g., PET measurements of regional blood flow and metabolism), studies have demonstrated profound stress-induced alterations within the same areas of the brain where major functional and pathologic changes occur in AD.

- The influence of various types of stress on immune function and brain metabolism has been reviewed by Plotnikoff et al (1992) in *Stress and Immunity*.

- Husband (1993) correlated life style, stress and disease—and associated changes involving hormones and neurotransmitters—in an extensive review of psychoimmunology.

- Concomitant biophysiologic aberrations relating to faulty diet, drastic alterations in work shifts, and potentially neurotoxic technological "advances"—factors discussed in previous chapters—are conducive to changes in nerve function. As a case in point, 17.8 percent of the nation's 80.5 million full-time workers work in shifts opposite to their natural sleep-wake cycle. Unchecked, these factors could culminate as AD or other degenerative brain disorders.

- The propriety of linking the nervous system and the immune system is further validated by the release of peptide neurotransmitters in Langerhans cells of the skin on exposure to a foreign substance, presumably to alert the immune system.

The influence of a high stress index on immunity is illustrated by the documented greater susceptibility to infection. A number of mechanisms are probably involved. They include impaired functioning of lymphocytes, and altered production of a number of neuroactive cytokines (including several interleukins and tumor necrosis factor) and hormones produced by the brain, pituitary, adrenal glands, and the immune system (Klein 1993).

- Experiments with animals have demonstrated their increased susceptibility to bacteria and viruses in response to various laboratory stressors (forced exercise;

120

restraint; isolation; avoidance learning; exposure to extremes of cold and heat).

- The vulnerability of frequent long-distance fliers to pneumonia and other infections (Brody 1993) suggests the immune-suppressing effects of travel-related stress, as well as poor-quality recirculation of cabin air (Chapter 12).

- The activation of certain cells (astrocytes, microglia) by cytokines within the brain can result in profound changes. They include behavioral disturbances, dementia and the destruction of neurons in the hippocampus and hypothalamus (Reichlin 1993).

- The influence of severe stress on immune function is illustrated by impaired lymphocyte reactivity among relatives of AD patients and residents in the area of the Three Mile Island nuclear disaster (Reichlin 1993).

THE EFFECTS OF STRESS

The psychological and physical benefits of inner peace, and the association of health with optimism and happiness, have been repeatedly affirmed. By contrast, pessimism and unhappiness tend to aggravate both organic and "functional" disorders, largely through neurotransmitter dysfunction (Chapter 5).

- Stress can reduce the number of serotonin receptors within the brain, especially in conjunction with depression (see below).

- The metabolic effects of stress are shown by significant elevations of the blood glucose, plasma lactic acid, and the heart rate in crying children (Aono 1993).

- Stressful medical disorders that create severe emotional upsets clearly contribute to mortality. For example, major depression following hospitalization for a heart attack (myocardial infarction) is a significant risk factor for mortality at six months (Frasure-Smith 1993).

The views of some students of stress differ from those expressed by Selye and others concerning certain aspects of its biological effects. However, there is general agreement that persons subjected to different forms of acute and chronic stress do manifest a general syndrome of ill health... even in the absence of demonstrable disease. It tends to be characterized by disturbances involving appetite, digestion, sleep, respiration, thermoregulation, and sexual desire.

> There is considerable current research on "the biology of fear," especially relative to subsequent depression and anxiety in the post-traumatic stress disorder. Animal studies underscore the centrality of the amygdala (a dense cluster of nerve fibers near the hippocampus) in the fear response.

Stress and Memory

Severe and prolonged stress can affect memory. The striking loss of memory during marked stress and depression may be evidenced as transient global amnesia, presumably due to "overloaded nerve circuits" within the brain.

- Dr. Joseph D. Sapira (1977), a respected medical educator, described his repeated encounter of impaired mentation afflicting medical students and young physicians under stress. (This disorder also affects high achievers in other professional groups.) Such turmoil often came in the wake of nonprofessional challenges of a geographic, family or social nature (e.g., a recent move, or the death of a parent). These doctors complained of marked difficulty in remembering medical reports they had recently read, and a sense of having lost control in the realm of patient care. It is not primarily a depression-type affective disorder, however, because the prognosis is usually good with supportive counsel.

- A resident of besieged Sarajevo provided a striking instance. This respected journalist in her mid-30s was interviewed during February 1993 as bombing of the city continued. She expressed amazement over the marked deterioration of her memory —for example, repeated inability to recall the day of the week.

- Salganik and Korczyn (1990) noted the increased risk of dementia patients with Parkinson's disease who had been subjected to the Holocaust.

Robert M. Sapolsky (1992) reviewed this subject in *Stress, the Aging Brain, and the Mechanisms of Neuron Death*. He hypothesized that adrenal hormones not only influence the brain, but can injure hippocampal neurons when released during chronic stress and in response to such noxious influences as hypoxia and alcohol—chiefly by (1) increasing their sensitivity to ischemia and excitatory neurotoxins, and (2) from excessive intracellular calcium rendering dying neurons unable to produce enough cellular energy in the form of adenosine triphosphate (ATP) to pump the calcium out of cells. These stimuli also release excess cortisone-like substances (glucocorticoids), resulting in "glucocorticoid endangerment." Elevated levels of glucocorticoids enhance neuronal damage from excitotoxins such as kainic acid. (The therapeutic role of glucocorticoid administration in accelerating brain aging for humans remains controversial.)

The impact of chronic stress on aging of the brain was raised in 1968 by Bruce McEwen of Rockefeller University. He noted the unusual vulnerability of the hippocampus, which is importantly involved in short-term memory, to diverse insults. This area contains many corticosterone receptors.

Tangle-like changes observed within the hippocampus in response to kainic acid are exacerbated by corticosterone (Mattson 1993).

INCREASED STRESSFULNESS IN CONTEMPORARY SOCIETY

Some will argue against the legitimacy of regarding stress as a risk factor for AD on the ground that severe anxiety from multiple threats has beset every previous generation. There is an element of uniqueness, however, about ongoing personal and societal upheavals during the 20th Century (see Introduction to Section I). Relentless confrontation with stressors are coupled with extraordinary rapidity of change, and uncertainty-insecurity from living and working in a highly complex and competitive society.

The 1993 World Labor Report by the International Labor Organization of the United Nations stated, "Stress has become one of the most serious health issues of the 20th Century." It regarded job stress as a "global phenomenon." Indeed, the Japanese have coined a term for death by overwork: karoshi.

- Stress-related diseases (e.g., peptic ulcer, hypertension, heart attacks) cost the United States economy $200 billion a year in absenteeism, compensation claims and medical expenses.

- Stress claims by government workers in Australia increased 90 percent in three years.

- Blue-collar workers tend to suffer more from job stress than their white-collar counterparts because they work in harsher environments and are paid less.

- Working women in most countries tend to suffer more from stress than men when they assume duties that involve both job and family.

Stress also tends to become a "circular" ailment (Dart 1993). Workers who encounter it at work and during arduous commuting often release their tensions on returning home… thereby creating a vicious cycle.

Workers and others who are "plugged in" to computers face electronic monitoring and newer unforeseen pressures. Consider the enormous impact of *information overload* created by the computer revolution. Millions of pieces of information and advertising incessantly assault the population, often in tiny time fragments (e.g., on television). Information overload is likely to increase exponentially with the advent of increasingly complex and rapidly changing "interactive media" spawned by so-called electronic superhighways that use hundreds of interacting channels and multimedia combinations.

- Children now appear to process information more quickly than their parents, a characteristic attributed to constant bombardment with disparate images (Cooper 1993). It is reflected in their language and "sound-byting of data," especially the jargon of contemporary slang. However, there is a price—as reflected in their limited patience for speeches and explanations that are not peppered with snappy phrases.

- Based on statistics from the Library of Congress, it is estimated that as many words are published <u>every week</u> as the total number of words published up to the year 1800.

- More than 5,000 new articles are published <u>daily</u> in the medical literature! This phenomenon generates much anxiety among physicians, even those who recently completed their training. One consequence has been the emphasis on specialization within limited areas.

- ERS-1, the European Earth-observing satellite which emits data equivalent to 2,500 copies of the Encyclopedia Britannica each day (*Science* August 13, 1993, p. 847), provides another example of data overload.

Then there is "urgency addiction" stemming from *"the hurry disease"* (Chapter 19), with emphasis on "time management." Some manifestations are the appeal of "sound bytes," "instant food," and abstracts of abstracts.

CONSEQUENCES OF PROLONGED STRESS

The long-term consequences of constant or repeated intense assaults on brain function and the human spirit are encountered daily in medical practice. They contribute to depression, panic attacks, chronic fatigue, compulsiveness, drug abuse, alcoholism, marriage problems, work addiction, and even suicide. Brief perusal of the yellow pages in a telephone directory will reveal "hot lines" for alcoholism, other forms of drug abuse, runaways, gamblers, rape, sexually-transmitted diseases, and abuse of women, children and the elderly.

McEwen and Stellar (1993) emphasized "the hidden cost of chronic stress" over prolonged periods, especially in individuals more susceptible to stress. They underscore the phenomenon of the <u>allostatic load</u>. This refers to the toll of chronic exposure to fluctuating or heightenened neural-neuroendocrine responses to repeated environmental challenges viewed as stressful.

Depression

The 20th Century has been viewed as ushering in the Age of Anxiety, and exiting as the Age of Melancholy. An international study indicates that major depression continues to increase worldwide… each successive generation appearing more vulnerable, especially young persons (Goleman 1992). Indeed, they are estimated to be three times more likely to experience intense depression than their grandparents' generation.

Studies of this epidemic have invoked various contributory factors. They include the stresses of industrialization, the loss of religious faith, unreasonable ideals of feminine beauty, and exposure to chemical neurotoxins.

The subject of depression as a risk factor in AD will be discussed further in Chapters 16 and 19.

Effects on Children

An extraordinary decade-long study by Stevenson et al (1993) attempted to determine the mathematics achievement of Chinese, Japanese and American children. It unexpectedly showed the considerable stress manifested by American eleventh graders. This finding surfaced as a result of asking students about the frequency with which they experienced feelings of stress, depression, aggression, sleeping difficulty, and somatic complaints—especially relative to academic anxiety. Seventy percent of the American students acknowledged such stresses, partly as the result of considerable more dating and working after school. (These observations also indicate the fallacy of a Western stereotype of Asian students as being more tense because of relentless pressure by parents to achieve academic excellence.)

Stress and Cerebrovascular Disease

Stress can contribute to the dementia resulting from "small strokes" (multi-infarct dementia) in several ways—most notably as a factor aggravating hypertension and elevated cholesterol levels. There also is evidence that anger, aggression and other components of Type A behavior (Chapter 19) correlate with plaque formation ("hardening of the arteries") in the carotid arteries that carry blood to the brain (Matsumoto 1993).

Attitudes Concerning Senility

Another undermining psychologic factor is the widespread pessimistic attitude toward "senility," based on the false premise that it is a predestined state. This idea can contribute to a vicious cycle of inappropriate worry, anger, resentment, boredom, the inability to love, and "old thinking."

SECTION III

RISK FACTORS FOR ALZHEIMER'S DISEASE

*For there is nothing covered that shall not be revealed;
neither hid, that shall not be known.*

Luke (12:2)

*Only by an aggressive approach to research and treatment [of
Alzheimer's disease] can we hope to help those currently
suffering from the disease and alter the fate of
those not yet afflicted.*

Alzheimer's Association Task Force

*Long-delayed effects are frequently difficult to relate to their
specific causes. Thus, it is conceivable that injuries due to
unrecognized causes have been produced by common
materials that have long been considered safe as
food or for use in foods. In this regard we are
concerned with cancer, genetic damage
and birth defects, premature and old age,
cardiovascular, endocrine and mental
disorders, and other human ills
of unexplained etiology.**

Julius M. Coon (1970)

---

*©1970 *Modern Medicine*. Reproduced with permission.

14

A LISTING OF RISK FACTORS; ILLUSTRATIVE CASE HISTORIES

The fact that it's difficult to see the signs doesn't necessarily mean that they don't exist. The signs are there to be seen, if we could understand them.

Mark van Doren

We have multitudes of facts, but we require, as they accumulate, organizations of them into higher knowledge; we require generalizations and working hypotheses.

Hughlings Jackson
(Pioneer neurologist)

I presented an hypothesis about the multifactorial causation of Alzheimer's disease (AD), and the supporting evidences, in previous chapters. The concept of multiple risk factors, both major ("primary") and minor ("contributory"; "permissive"), is consistent with the view that AD represents a "convergence syndrome" (Blass 1993).

Clues to the existence of neurotoxic influences and other "risk factors" often can be detected or inferred during the decades of "early" or "transitional" AD. They are derived from one's family history, personal habits, exposure to known neurotoxins in the home and work environments, previous medical and surgical illnesses, the physical examination, and various testing methods (exclusive of those used to exclude other causes of dementia.)

126

The importance of "the infinitely little" in diagnosis was stressed by Dr. Joseph Bell, whom many regard as the "real" Sherlock Holmes. In his essay, "In Praise of Dr. Doyle" (December 1892 issue of *The Bookman*), Bell stated: "Racial peculiarities, hereditary tricks of manner, accent, occupation or the want of it, education, environment of all kinds, by their little trivial impressions gradually mould or carve the individual, and leave finger marks or chisel scores which the expert can recognize... There are myriads of signs eloquent and instructive, but which need the educated eye to detect."

The detection of risk factors or "early warning signals" for AD would seem a prerequisite before initiating long-term preventive or therapeutic measures in individuals perceived to be vulnerable... and long before any hint of a dementing process. This concept has counterparts in conventional medical practice, such as preventive recommendations for coronary heart disease, diabetes mellitus and several cancers— based on accepted risk factors for these diseases.

I list below various influences that appear to favor or accelerate AD. The location of relevant discussions in previous chapters is noted, as well as pertinent references. An asterisk (*) indicates a perceived "major" risk factor, based on prolonged personal observation of patients and current knowledge. Experimental laboratory tests will be omitted, notwithstanding their considerable interest.

The summaries of several patients with AD and in the AD-prone state follow. They indicate how such information can be made operational within the clinical setting.

PREVIOUS STUDIES

Many investigators have tried to identify risk factors for AD. Their fine efforts remain of limited value, however, largely because of failure to encompass the panorama of likely causative and contributory influences.

The Ramsey Foundation Brain Bank

Mendez et al (1991) analyzed the clinical and pathologic data of the Ramsey Foundation Brain Bank. Clinical questionnaires were completed by the families and caregivers of 407 AD patients. The records of 100 patients having dementia due to other causes, and of 50 normal elderly subjects, served as controls.

The only statistically significant finding was a positive family history of AD affecting a first-degree relative in 134 (33 percent). Other possible risk factors included heart disease (33 percent), hypertension (25 percent), clinical cerebral vascular disease (20 percent), a history of head trauma (16 percent), abuse of alcohol (9.3 percent), and thyroid disease (7 percent).

Review of More Than 50 General Population Surveys of Dementia by the National Health and Medical Research Council of Australia (Henderson 1990)

The chief findings derived from these studies were the exponential increase of dementia with age (i.e., the rates doubling every 5.1 years), and the higher AD rates among women. The significance of a wide variation in prevalence rates could not be determined.

This group sought risk factors for AD among 11 case-control studies. It encompassed 1,294 AD patients and 1,353 control subjects.

- AD accounted for two-thirds of cases having global dementia.

- There was a strong association between AD and a family history of dementia.

- There was a strong association between AD and Down's syndrome (mongolism).

- An association between AD and a family history of Parkinson's disease could be shown.

- A history of depression increased the risk for AD.

- The risk for AD nearly doubled when previous head trauma had been associated with loss of consciousness.

Rochester Population-Based Case-Control Study (Kokmen et al 1991)

This population-based case-control study of AD involved Rochester (Minnesota) residents. Episodic depression, a personality disorder, and hypertension were the only statistically significant features found among the more than 20 possible clinical risk factors evaluated.

RESERVATIONS AND LIMITATIONS

In view of the inherent limitations of this approach, the following qualifiers are appropriate.

- The relative contribution of "nature" and "nurture" may not be clear when relatives have been afflicted with AD. Repeated mention was made of possible exposure to culturally-influenced neurotoxins involving persons living in the same household.

- Persons having one or several risk factors might never develop AD during their life span even though changes in the brain (e.g., neurofibrillary tangles) do exist.

- Extended epidemiologic studies concerning benefits of the preventive regimen set forth in Chapters 17-19 will be required—in part because AD-prone persons who adhere to it may never manifest dementia or another degenerative neurologic disorder.

An additional disclaimer for physicians and health professionals should be emphasized. As repeatedly noted, they must "THINK ALZHEIMER'S!" when encountering patients with multiple risk factors and atypical symptoms. On the other hand, *extreme caution* should be exercised before making a formal diagnosis of "early AD" or "proneness to AD" because an emotional upheaval might be precipitated.

This contrasts with conveying the diagnosis of "probable Alzheimer's disease" (PAD) on the basis of features described in Chapter 1. Such information could be crucial for a patient who is still capable of making informed decisions, and of formulating advanced directives before the condition progresses to the point where gross dementia would preclude doing so.

A LISTING OF POSSIBLE RISK FACTORS FOR ALZHEIMER'S DISEASE

(* indicates a probable "major" risk factor)

I. Family History

- Medical and Neurological Illnesses

    Dementia ("senile"; "presenile") (see above) (Chapter 3)*

    Down's syndrome (mongolism; trisomy 21) (see above)*

    Parkinson's disease (see above) (Chapter 15)*

    Amyotrophic lateral sclerosis (Chapter 15)*

    Hypoglycemia ("low blood sugar attacks") (Chapter 8)*

    Phenylketonuria (PKU) (Chapter 9)

    Reactions to aspartame (NutraSweet®) products (Chapter 9)*

    Narcolepsy (Chapter 15)*

    Hyperactivity (Chapter 15)*

    Multiple sclerosis (Chapter 15)

    Galactosemia (Chapter 9)

    Parental history of diabetes and hypertension (see above)

    (Wing 1992)

- Racial Propensity to Functional (Diabetogenic) Hyperinsulinism (Chapters 8)*

    Jews

    Italians

    African Americans

    Native Americans (Indians)

- Advanced maternal age (Chapter 16)

    Especially when nausea and vomiting persisted throughout the pregnancy

II. Past History

- Excessive birth weight (greater than 8 pounds) (Chapters 8 and 16)
- Very-low-birth weight (see above) (Chapters 7 and 8)*
- Neonatal hypoglycemia (Chapter 8)*
- "Colic" in infants, with associated nocturnal crying and excessive irritability
- Hyperactivity (Chapter 15)*
- Depression (Hoffman 1991) (see above) (Chapter 16)*

- Migraine (Chapter 15)*
- "Minimal brain dysfunction"; "attention deficit syndrome"; reading disability (Chapter 16)*
- Seizures in childhood*
- Thyroid disease (Chapter 16)*
- Severe malnutrition (Chapter 7)*
- Marked fluctuations in weight (Chapters 7 and 16)
- Intolerance to products containing aspartame (Chapter 9)*
- Intolerance to monosodium glutamate (MSG) and hydrolyed vegetable protein (HVP)(Chapter 9)*
- Adverse reactions to the prolonged use of oral contraceptives ("the pill") (Chapter 8)
- Large intake of aluminum-containing antacids for gastrointestinal or kidney disorders (Chapter 10)*
- History of general anesthesia, especially when prolonged and multiple (Chapter 11)*
- Head injury ("dementia pugilistica") (Chapter 16)*
- Low educational attainment (Chapter 16)

III. Habits and Exposures

- Excessive and prolonged intake of sugar (Chapters 7 and 8)*
- Excessive intake of high-fructose corn syrup (Chapter 8)*
- Prolonged smoking (Chapter 12)*
- Alcohol abuse (Mendez 1991)*
- Considerable intake of the food additives aspartame and MSG (Chapter 9)*
- Preference for excessively heated meat ("well done"; barbecued) (Chapter 7)
- Considerable intake of "gourmet" foods (Chapter 9)
- Chronic use of appetite-suppressing drugs (selective damage to neurotransmitter nerve cells and pathways) (Chapter 11)
- Vigorous dieting with repeated weight loss (Chapters 7 and 16)*
- Considerable intake of aluminum (e.g., antacids; habitual tea drinking) (Chapter 10)*
- Exposure to lead (e.g., paint; hair dyes) (Chapter 11)*
- Exposure to mercury (e.g., multiple amalgam fillings) (Chapter 11)*
- Use of fluoridated water, toothpaste and mouthwashes (Chapter 11)
- Prolonged use of oral contraceptives ("the pill"), especially by women over 40 (Winslow 1991)*
- Abuse of drugs (prescription; illicit) (Chapter 11)*
- Use of inhalants to achieve "a high" (Chapter 11)

- Severe electric shock injury (occupational; home) (Roberts 1966f)
- Longstanding proximity to power lines and large antennas (Chapter 16)
- Exposure to carbon monoxide (Chapters 11 and 12)*

  Cigarette smoking

  A major fire

  Prolonged air travel in newer large aircraft with reduced air recirculation (Tolchin 1993)
- Frequent and extended viewing of movies and television (Chapter 16)
- Extended working on night shifts (Chapter 16)
- Habitual wearing of sunglasses (Chapter 16)

IV. Clinical Features and Complications of Severe Hypoglycemia*

(Chapters 8 and 16)

- Reactive hypoglycemia ("low blood sugar") attacks
- Disorders related to, or aggravated by, hypoglycemia

  Severe leg cramps at night (Roberts 1965a, 1973)

  "Restless legs" (Roberts 1965a, 1973)

  Peripheral neuropathies

  The narcolepsy complex (narcolepsy; intensely vivid dreams, sleep paralysis; cataplexy) (Roberts 1964, 1967b, 1971b) (Chapter 15)

  Unexplained chronic fatigue (Chapter 16)

  Unexplained seizures, especially at night (Roberts 1964, 1971b)

  Unexplained angina pectoris or cardiac arrhythmias, especially at night (Roberts 1967a, 1991b)

  Unexplained labyrinthine ("inner ear") attacks

  Migraine and related vascular headaches (Chapter 15)

  Prostatic hypertrophy (Roberts 1966a, 1967c)

  Thyropathies (goiter; hyperthyroidism; hypothyroidism) (Roberts 1969a) (Chapter 16)
- Diabetes mellitus

  Children (Holmes 1987)

  Adults with recurrent insulin reactions (Holmes 1987)
- Episodic depression (Kokmen 1991) (Chapter 16)
- Unexplained driving accidents (Gilley 1991) (Chapter 1)

V. Physical Findings

- Age (Chapter 1)*

- Female gender (Chapter 16)
- Skin "markers" for the syndrome of hypoglycemia and narcolepsy (Roberts 1964, 1965c, 1971b)

  Café au lait spots

  Localized hypomelanosis

  Atypical melanin pigmentation

  Supernumerary nipple

  Occipital or lumbar nevus

- Excessive weight (Roberts 1967b)
- Intentional severe weight loss (including anorexia nervosa) (Chapter 16)*
- Excessive height (more than 6 feet) (Chapter 16)*
- Cataracts before the age of 60
- Hyperactivity (Chapter 15)*
- "Benign essential tremor" (Chapter 15)*
- Hypertension (Chapter 16)*

VI. Laboratory Clues

- "Reactive" hypoglycemia and decreased glucose tolerance by glucose tolerance testing, with concomitant excess insulin release (Chapter 8)*
- Hypothyroidism (especially elevated TSH level) (Chapter 16)*
- Excessive deposition of toxic metals—aluminum, lead, mercury; arsenic; thallium—by hair analysis and other methods (Chapter 11)*
- Studies indicating a carrier state for phenylketonuria and galactosemia (Chapter 9)
- Prior or concomitant asymptomatic cerebral disease detected by imaging studies (normal-pressure hydrocephalus; post-trauma injury)*
- Hippocampal atrophy by magnetic resonance imaging (MRI) studies (Scheltens 1991, Kesslak 1991) (Chapters 1 and 4)*

  May constitute a biological marker that precedes the symptoms of AD (de Leon et al 1993)

- Imaging studies (PET; SPECT) evidencing focal reduction of glucose uptake (Panchalingham 1991) (Chapter 8)*
- Apolipoprotein E type 4 (apoE4) associated with plasma lipoproteins (Chapter 3)*

REPRESENTATIVE CASE HISTORIES

I commented earlier on the importance of long-term observation for uncovering AD risk factors. The review of patients who were attended *many years before* AD was even considered affirms this point.

Several patients summarized below indicate how such insights can be made operational in the trenches of medical practice. The more relevant details appear in italics.

The first patient illustrates both the existence of multiple prior risk factors, and the subtle evolution of AD over several decades. Her two sisters with comparable risk factors were probably evidencing transitional AD.

CASE 1

A 51 year-old housewife was seen for *hypoglycemic attacks* that occurred when she did not eat for three hours or longer. A morning glucose tolerance test revealed *decreased glucose tolerance* (elevated blood glucose concentrations after ingesting the glucose load), followed by reactive hypoglycemia. There was striking improvement when she avoided sugar and took small snacks.

The patient also was found to have an *underactive thyroid (hypothyroidism)*. This condition improved on Synthroid® therapy.

She later experienced recurrent episodes of pancreatitis, the first during January 1974. She ingested *considerable aluminum* containing antacids for this condition, and later for a symptomatic hiatal hernia with esophageal reflux.

A barium enema was recommended by another doctor when she was 58. Rapid palpitations and extreme confusion due to hypoglycemia occurred after abstaining from food in preparation for this examination. Brief hospitalization was required.

When seen eight months later, her *confusion and memory loss* had progressed. Other complaints included *intermittent unsteadiness and headaches*. Multiple CT scans of the head proved normal.

The *surgical and anesthesia history* were pertinent. A hysterectomy had been done at the age of 38 for uterine fibroids. The patient underwent removal of the gallbladder in 1970, cataract surgery in 1972, and partial resection of the colon for recurrent diverticulitis in 1982. She also received many *local infiltrations with a local anesthetic (lidocaine)* for bursitis and tendinitis.

The patient was *allergic or intolerant to a number of drugs*. Her breasts became tender from vitamin E and Premarin.® She intermittently used tranquilizers and sedatives, primarily Librium® and Elavil®.

In July 1986, she complained of *increased confusion, intense headache, marked fatigue, unsteadiness,* severe *insomnia* (i.e., awakening during the night), repeated "cracking" of the ears, pain in the eyes, and atypical pains over the left chest and shoulder. Other symptoms included *"severe nervousness," depression, and intolerance to noise.* Direct questioning revealed that she had been drinking much *tea sweetened with aspartame* for several months. Furthermore, her husband made an aspartame-sweetened chocolate pudding and homemade ice cream with considerable aspartame in an attempt to avoid sugar. The diagnosis of *aspartame reactor* was confirmed when these complaints subsided after avoiding such products… including the ability to communicate without needing notes.

By September 1990, she evidenced a *parkinsonian tremor* and further memory loss. The diagnosis of probable Alzheimer's disease was made independently by a psychiatric consultant. Subsequent nuclear SPECT brain imaging and cerebral flow studies revealed temporal lobe deficits consistent with "a mild or early Alzheimer's pattern."

SISTER OF CASE 1

This sister was 60 when seen in consultation during April 1981. She complained of severe sweats and foot-leg cramps during the night. There was intermittent burning of the toes. She had taken Dyazide® for *hypertension.* A diagnosis of probable *lactase deficiency* was made on the basis of marked gas and indigestion after drinking milk. There were *allergies* to aspirin, penicillin, lidocaine, sulfonamides and intravenous dyes.

The diagnosis of *reactive hypoglycemia due to functional hyperinsulinism* was confirmed by morning glucose tolerance testing. The results were as follows:

	Blood Glucose (mg%)	Blood Insulin (μU/ml)
Fasting	100	41
1/2 hour	141	351
1 hour	140	174
2 hours	151	260
3 hours	131	—
4 hours	96	—
4 1/2 hours	59*	—

(* - clinical hypoglycemic attack)

Several studies indicated the presence of *hypothyroidism.* Her son also had hypothyroidism.

The patient used *considerable hair dye and underarm deodorant.* The results of hair analysis indicated 2.1 parts per million (ppm) of *mercury* (upper limit of normal), and 11 ppm *aluminum.*

When seen in June 1984, she complained of *marked deterioration in her ability to remember names.* A random blood sugar concentration was only 62 mg%. It was ascertained that *she had resisted taking the recommended feedings during the mid-afternoon and before retiring in spite of experiencing severe hunger.*

ANOTHER SISTER OF CASE 1

This sister was 75 when seen in October 1984 for long-standing *hypoglycemic attacks.* She *predictably developed severe confusion, lightheadedness, tremor and hunger several hours after eating sugar or sweets.* Oranges also precipitated attacks. Other symptoms included *severe leg cramps* during the night, and *marked numbness or burning of the feet.* She was *intolerant to aspirin.*

The physical examination revealed a *decline of the systolic blood pressure on standing* (from 130 mm Hg to 110 mm Hg), and *diminished ankle jerks.* A random blood glucose was 60 mg%. The results of a morning glucose tolerance test indicated elevated glucose levels at 3 and 3-1/2 hours, and increased insulin concentrations that persisted for two hours after the glucose load. The study was terminated at 4-1/2 hours when she experienced a severe hypoglycemic attack.

The patient subsequently volunteered that there was considerable improvement after adhering to an appropriate diet and supportive measures.

She required an emergency visit one year later for *severe headache, a profound loss of memory,* weakness, and other complaints after having gone seven hours without eating. A CT scan of the brain was normal. Her symptoms subsided within several days after resuming the recommended diet and snacks.

15

ASSOCIATED OR RELATED NEUROLOGIC DISORDERS

*The line between nutritional insult and measurable effect in terms of
health may be quite long. A period of 40 or more years may elapse
before a secondary manifestation occurs. Such is thought to be
the case in Parkinson's syndrome characterized by
neurological tremors and progressive rigidity of
limbs, trunk and face.*

C. Edith Weir (1971, p.53)

*Before concluding these pages, it may be proper to observe once
more that an important object proposed to be obtained by them
is the leading of the attention of those who humanely employ
anatomical examination in detecting the cause and nature of
diseases, particularly to this malady. By their benevolent
labours its real nature may be ascertained,and appropriate
modes of relief, or even of cure, pointed out.*

James Parkinson (1817)

I have indicated that Alzheimer's disease (AD) represents one type of reaction by
the brain to injury from multiple insults—nutritional; hypoxemic; neurotoxic—that are
prevalent in our society (Chapters 4 and 6). It therefore should not come as a surprise
that *other degenerative disorders of the nervous system may be caused or influenced by
similar exposures and overlapping mechanisms.* (The term "degenerative" refers to the
shriveling and disappearance of cells in the absence of inflammation or an interrupted
blood supply).

136

Furthermore, *several of these neurologic conditions may precede or accompany AD*—e.g., migraine; seizures; narcolepsy; Parkinson's disease. The latter also is characterized by a long period before the onset of severe tremor and stiffness, during which there might be intermittent nonmotor features (Koller 1992). The associations of AD with depression, chronic fatigue and head trauma are discussed in Chapter 16.

Some of these neurologic features can appear many years before the clinical onset of dementia. Accordingly, they should be regarded as possible risk factors and early warning clues for proneness to AD (Chapter 14)... and signals to institute the preventive measures described in Section IV.

Hypoglycemia ("low blood sugar attacks") due to "functional" hyperinsulinism (Chapter 8) constitutes an important common metabolic denominator in the causation and aggravation of important neurologic disorders other than AD. I have described its major role in migraine (Roberts 1967d), epileptic seizures (Roberts 1964 a,b, 1971b), narcolepsy (Roberts 1964 a,b,c, 1967b, 1969b, 1971b), reading disability (Roberts 1969b), restless legs and other muscle disorders (Roberts 1965a, 1973), and multiple sclerosis (Roberts 1966 b,c).

MIGRAINE HEADACHES

The dramatic increase of migraine in the past decade overlaps with that of AD. Its averaged prevalence per 1,000 population—for both men and women—rose from 25.8 per 1,000 population in 1980 to 41 per 1,000 population in 1989 (Centers for Disease Control 1991).

Several of the metabolic, hypoxemic and neurotoxic mechanisms associated with migraine may initiate comparable changes in evolving AD.

- The spasm of arteries in migraine reduces oxygen to the brain (Chapter 12), and releases neurotoxic excitatory amino acids, especially glutamate (Ferrari 1990) (Chapter 9).

- Hypoglycemia (Chapter 8) <u>frequently</u> precipitates migraine (Roberts 1967d).

- Abnormalities in the mitochondria (intracellular structures involved with energy) (Chapter 8) have been shown in patients having prolonged migrainous auras (sensations preceding the headache attack) and migraine-associated strokes (Montagna 1988).

- Montagna et al (1994) demonstrated metabolic abnormalities of the brain in persons with migraine <u>without</u> aura by ^{31}P-magnetic resonance spectroscopy. These subjects evidenced significantly low phosphocreatine, increased adenosine diphosphate and decreased phosphorylation potential—along with a slow rate of phosphocreatine recovery in muscle after exercise.

The high prevalence of migraine in a Peruvian population living 14,200 feet above sea level provides impressive evidence for the role of hypoxemia. Arregui et al (1991) reported a 12.4 percent rate there, compared to 3.6 percent in a sea-level population.

NARCOLEPSY (PATHOLOGIC DROWSINESS AND SLEEP)

My early studies on narcolepsy and related phenomena—namely, sleep paralysis, hallucinations before or after sleep, and loss of muscle tone (cataplexy)—have been detailed in prior publications (Roberts 1964, 1966, 1967, 1971). At that time, I did not recognize an association between narcolepsy and AD. This likely relationship subsequently became evident after observing such patients for prolonged periods.

Others have confirmed my impression about the prevalence of narcolepsy, especially relative to accident proneness (Roberts 1971b) and chronic "fatigue" (Chapter 16). The National Commission on Sleep Disorders Research reported that more than 40 millions Americans (!) have significant sleepiness—that is, to the point of either inviting danger or failing to live up to one's potential. The following observations were noted:

- Up to two-thirds of all drivers sometimes feel sleepy at the wheel. Ten percent of these dozed, and had been involved in at least one accident.
- Half of manufacturing workers on duty during night shifts sleep on the job at least once weekly.
- One-fourth of teenagers admit to falling asleep in school once a week.

The localization of changes within the locus ceruleus and other areas of the brain in both AD and narcolepsy lends added credence for such an association.

- The locus ceruleus, a small collection of nerve cells below the cerebral cortex, is intimately involved with norepinephrine neurotransmission within the brain (Chapter 5).
- Damage to the nucleus basalis of Meynert also occurs in AD. This area has been closely linked to impaired acetylcholine metabolism (Chapter 5).

I have emphasized that (1) adequate substrate for energy (chiefly from glucose) is required by the sleep centers, and (2) certain electroencephalographic responses (such cyclic REM activity) probably represent a compensatory mechanism when vital brain cells sense a reduction of available glucose (Roberts 1971b).

HYPERACTIVITY

Hypoglycemia contributes importantly to hyperactivity, both during childhood and adulthood (Roberts 1965a, 1969b, 1973). Moreover, reduced glucose metabolism by the brain—both global and in focal areas of the cortex—has been found in adults with "hyperactivity of childhood onset" by positron emission tomographic (PET) scanning (Zametkin 1990). The similar reduction of cerebral glucose metabolism in AD was reviewed in Chapter 8.

READING DISABILITY (DYSLEXIA) AND ATTENTION-DEFICIT DISORDER

The eventual risk for AD in children and young persons with reading disability (dyslexia) requires considerable study. I have reported the apparent fundamental role of hypoglycemia and poor nutrition in dyslexia (Roberts 1969b).

This association is bolstered by the inferred localization of such impairment within areas of the brain known to be more sensitive to glucose deprivation. As a case in point, PET scans reveal a smaller size of Broca's area in the left brain, which is responsible for processing rapid sensory signals (Tallal 1992).

There has been increased recognition of the fact that attention-deficit disorder (ADD) continues into adult life. An estimated 8-15 million American adults have this condition, including more than half of the prison population (Miller 1993). ADD is characterized by a short attention span (especially for low-interest activities), difficulty in listening, low frustration tolerance, argumentativeness, frequent mood swings, a tendency to avoid group activities, relative underachievement, procrastination, difficulty in completing tasks, forgetfulness, restlessness at night, and frequent job changes. It can be confused with anxiety and manic depression. ADD is believed to result from neurotransmitter dysfunction.

The familial aspects of ADD are noteworthy. In a number of instances, the making of this diagnosis in a child led to correct diagnosis of a parent—and the institution of appropriate measures (e.g., Ritalin®).

BENIGN (ESSENTIAL) TREMOR

So-called benign or essential tremor is encountered relatively frequently in medical practice. Several observations suggest that it may be an early clinical feature in patients who later develop AD or Parkinson's disease (see below). For example, parkinsonism was found in 20 percent of 350 patients who had essential tremor (Lou 1991).

PARKINSON'S DISEASE

Although several drugs are effective in the management of Parkinson's disease (PD), its cause remains as much a challenge as AD. Since PD and AD overlap clinically and experimentally in many respects (see below), it is reasonable to infer common causative mechanisms. Indeed, the increasing frequency of PD in younger persons could reflect the accordioned adverse effects of diet, environmental neurotoxins, and other factors. Dr. J. William Langston (1991), a pioneer in PD research, also believes that this disorder is primarily due to environmental rather than genetic influences.

As a corollary, similar precautionary measures (Section IV) could be beneficial in preventing or delaying both conditions.

Another Neurologic Continuum

The prolonged duration of "evolving" or "transitional" AD was discussed in Chapters 4 and 6. Similarly, PD probably begins a decade or more before the typical tremor and rigidity appear. This is consistent with (1) the detection of marked degeneration in the substantia nigra (the area of the brain predominantly affected), and (2) the loss therein of dopamine, the major neurotransmitter involved, during this transitional phase. Reduced striatal dopamine also has been shown by PET imaging in "at-risk" individuals.

The pathologic and clinical continuum of PD has counterparts in "early"

Alzheimer's disease (Chapter 6) and multiple sclerosis (Roberts 1966c). This view is shared by others.

- Koller (1992) referred to the decrease of "Parkinson's disease protective factor" and a "premorbid parkinsonian personality."

- Marsden (1990) suggested "preclinical Parkinson's disease" in a "large cohort of normal middle-aged and early individuals, who… if they live long enough, may get the disease in later life."

Common Denominators in Parkinsonism and Alzheimer's Disease

Significant clinical, laboratory and epidemiologic features in both PD and AD lend credence to the conviction that common mechanisms are probably operative.

- One of four patients with PD develops dementia (Brown 1984).

- A family history of PD represents a risk factor for AD (Hoffman 1991).

- There is more rapid progression of probable AD in patients who evidence features suggesting PD during their early symptomatic course (Mortimer 1992).

- One-third of patients with PD who receive long-term levodopa therapy develop dementia of the Alzheimer type.

- The amyotrophic lateral sclerosis-parkinsonism-dementia syndrome among Guamanian Chamorros who ingest a neurotoxin present in the Cycad plant constitutes another link.

- There is considerable overlap of the abnormalities by functional imaging studies in AD patients and patients with PD who develop dementia.

- The molecular nature of senile plaque proteins (Chapter 4) present in the hippocampus of PD patients and AD patients is similar (Arai 1992).

- Demented PD patients also have reduced choline acetyltransferase activity (Perry 1983) (Chapter 5).

- Many persons who experience reactions to aspartame products (Chapter 9) not only develop marked confusion and memory loss but also severe tremor (Roberts 1989a). Indeed, the diagnosis of PD was often considered before the tremor regressed when these products were avoided.

- Hypoglycemia due to functional (diabetogenic) hyperinsulinism frequently occurs in patients with AD (Chapter 8) and PD. The nadir responses by PD patients given oral glucose (100 gm) (Boyd 1971) are also consistent with reactive hypoglycemia.

16

OTHER POSSIBLE RISK FACTORS

More is missed by not looking than by not knowing.

Thomas Moore

A careful physician… before he attempts to administer a remedy to his patient, must investigate not only the malady of the man he wishes to cure, but also his habits when in health and his physical constitution.

Cicero
(On the Orator)

Numerous clinical hints concerning increased vulnerability of the brain are detectable during the long "transitional" phase of Alzheimer's disease (AD) (Chapter 6); some may be traceable to childhood and early adult life. There is an analogy in this respect to the multiple-sclerosis-prone state (Roberts 1966b,c).

Doctors should "THINK ALZHEIMER'S!" when atypical or unexplained neuropsychiatric complaints and other pertinent features are encountered, especially among persons having multiple risk factors (Chapter 14). The conditions and considerations discussed below and in Chapter 15 could have considerable value if they identify susceptibility to this affliction.

DEPRESSION AND OTHER PSYCHIATRIC DISORDERS

The dramatic rise of depression during the latter part of the 20th Century (Chapter 13) is a worldwide problem (Goleman 1992). Those who have investigated this phenomenon regard it as the culmination of many factors and stresses, including exposure to neurotoxic substances. Dr. Thomas Szasz (1991) provided this pertinent perspective: "If mental illnesses are diseases of the central nervous system, they are diseases of the brain, not of mind."

The only neurologic or psychiatric disorders significantly associated with AD in a population-based case-controlled study of Rochester (Minnesota) residents were a history of personality disorder and episodic depression (Kokmen 1991).

These observations are germane:

- Patients with prior pseudodementia (Chapter 1) can develop true dementia (Kral 1989).

- The decreased metabolism of certain brain areas in depressed patients as found by PET studies on (Mayberg 1992)—notably the basitemporal limbic pathways—provides more evidence for such an interrelation.

- Depression may occur a decade or longer before the overt onset of Parkinson's disease (PD) (Koller 1992) (Chapter 15).

- Marder et al (1993) concluded that depressive symptoms independently predict the development of dementia in PD patients.

ATYPICAL MANIFESTATIONS OF HYPOGLYCEMIA AND DIABETES

(Chapter 8)

Most physicians are not aware of the major role played by severe hypoglycemia in a number of conditions involving the central and peripheral nervous systems, with or without diabetes. Reference to these disorders was made previously. They are again listed as possible epiphenomena of "early" AD.

- Vascular headaches (Roberts 1967d)

- Epilepsy in its various forms (Roberts 1964a,b)

- Narcolepsy (Roberts 1964a,b; 1967, 1971b)

- Multiple sclerosis (Roberts 1966b,c)

- Learning disability (Roberts 1969b)

- Peripheral neuropathy, including postural hypotension (Roberts 1982a)

- Restless legs (Roberts 1965a, 1972)

- Psychiatric dysfunction (Roberts 1964)

- Behavioral disturbances (Roberts 1971b)

Metabolic and epidemiologic studies also suggest a relationship between AD and "functional" hyperinsulinism or diabetes mellitus.

- A positive association between AD and diabetes mellitus has been reported (McWhorter 1987).

- Higher circulating insulin levels were found in AD patients who did not have clinical diabetes (Adolfsson 1980).

- Harik and Kalaria (1992) noted a marked decrease (about 50 percent) in the density of the glucose transporter (Chapter 8) within isolated brain microvessels from AD patients.

THE "CHRONIC FATIGUE SYNDROME"

Fatigue is a frequent complaint that leads to medical attention, particularly by women and persons in the higher socioeconomic brackets. This complaint assumes considerable pertinence because *many individuals who develop AD had previously sought help for unexplained severe "fatigue."*

Persistent or relapsing fatigue admittedly poses many diagnostic and therapeutic changes. I reviewed them earlier (Roberts 1958, 1964c,3, 1966e, 1992d)—with emphasis upon unrecognized narcolepsy (Chapter 15) and reactive hypoglycemia (Chapter 8).

> The chronic fatigue syndrome has been referred to by many labels. One century ago, Julius Althaus, consultant physician at the Hospital for Epilepsy and Paralysis in London, wrote a new edition of *On Failure of Brain Power (Encephalasthenia); Its Nature and Treatment.* The numerous hypotheses for this disorder and advocated treatments over subsequent generations have been predicated on changes in brain function and architecture involving neurotransmitters, the limbic system and psychoneuroimmunology.

Cognitive disturbances involving memory and attention have been encountered in patients with the chronic fatigue syndrome. Objective changes also may be demonstrable.

- Natelson et al (1993) reported that patients with the chronic fatigue syndrome had significantly more abnormal MRI scans than controls. They recommended close followup of this subset of patients because "they may evolve more specific neurologic diagnoses."

- Weiger (1993) pointed out the demonstration of changes by MRI studies in patients with the chronic fatigue syndrome consistent with swelling or demyelination.

Severe fatigue can reflect the recurring impact on brain and bodily function of metabolic-hypoxemic disturbances, and of exposure to multiple neurotoxins. Indeed, several investigators have suggested a defect in oxidative metabolism involving skeletal muscles as a basis for the chronic fatigue syndrome.

> Wong et al (1992) studied 22 such patients by ^{31}P nuclear magnetic resonance spectroscopy. This enabled minute-to-minute assessment of intracellular high-energy phosphate metabolism of the gastrocnemius muscles in the leg. Patients with chronic fatigue exhausted more rapidly than normal subjects, at which point intracellular concentrations of adenosine triphosphate (ATP) (Chapter 8) were reduced.

It also must be stressed that *the aggressive and prolonged administration of tranquilizers and sedatives to such individuals could aggravate evolving AD* (Chapter 11).

The following letter from a 45-year-old woman illustrates the need to "THINK ALZHEIMER'S!" in persons with unexplained and progressive "chronic fatigue."

September 14, 1993

Dear Dr. Roberts:

I recently read your book about the effects of aspartame, and want to thank you for writing it! I have discontinued all products containing aspartame, thanks to you. The data you presented about methyl alcohol convinced me!!

I also understand that you are an internist and specialize in difficult diagnoses; you wrote a book titled *Difficult Diagnosis: A Guide to The Interpretation of Severe Illness.*

I am sending you this FAX in the hopes that you might have an interest in my case. I have had extensive medical testing done here in _____ , at the Mayo Clinic in Jacksonville, and the Cleveland Clinic and University Hospitals in Ohio.

My medical problem is that of increasing LOSS OF ALERTNESS on A DAILY BASIS. This has been going on for a number of yeras. The only two diagnoses found so far are hypothyroidism and low adrenal reserve. I am on Synthroid 0.05 mg. a day for one year now, and recently had a slight abnormality in my cortisone levels and am now on 20 mg of cortisone acetate a day. However, even with both of these medications, my increasing fatigue or loss of alertness continues to decline, and I feel worse every day. I also have been tried on NUMEROUS antidepressants, but all of these have been a waste of time.

My symptoms feel like I am "rapidly aging"—that is, my alertness is rapidly decreasing. I continue to feel worse EVERY DAY. This obviously has affected my employment, my social life, hobbies etc. to the point I cannot keep up with people my age and even older. I am 45 years "young!"

HIGH BLOOD PRESSURE (HYPERTENSION)

A significant correlation between hypertension and the risk of developing AD has been reported (Kokmen 1991). Moreover, memory and attention impairment can be detected in about half of hypertensive patients (Fioravanti 1991).

Hypertension also constitutes a major factor in dementia resulting from multiple strokes (multi-infarct dementia).

144

THYROID DISORDERS

Some investigators have reported a higher frequency of thyroid disease (especially Hashimoto's thyroiditis and hypothyroidism) prior to or in association with AD (Heyman 1984, Mortimer 1990, Mendez 1991, Yoshimasu 1991). These relationships are pertinent for the following reasons:

- There is an increased incidence of thyroid disorders among patients with hypoglycemia due to functional hyperinsulinism (Chapter 8) and diabetes. This probably reflects a compensatory response by the thyroid gland to tissue depletion of energy.

- Hyperthyroidism and thyroiditis have been precipitated in patients with hypoglycemia who subjected themselves to severe caloric restriction (Roberts 1969a).

- Autoimmunity (Chapter 6) contributes to several thyroid diseases and degenerative neurologic disorders (e.g., amyotrophic lateral sclerosis; multiple sclerosis).

Thyroid hormone crucially influences the development and optimum function of the nervous system, especially during infancy. These effects may be mediated in part by nerve growth factor (Chapter 5). There also are tissue-specific nerve growth factor responses to thyroid hormone (Hayden 1992).

INFLUENCES DURING PREGNANCY

The impression exists that *either extreme of maternal age increases the risk for AD in the children of such pregnancies.* It is amplified by concomitant diabetes, hypertension, other medical problems, poor habits, and exposure to potential neurotoxins during pregnancy.

Long ago, Dr. Arnold Lorand (1910) observed that persons afflicted with premature old age may be "the victims of the immoderation of their ancestors" (p. 116). He urged pregnant women to avoid "anything that may prove fatal to the foetus or influence its nutrition"… especially the use of drugs.

A number of metabolic, hypoxemic and toxicologic influences during pregnancy are known to interfere with the crucial migration of neurons. They include alcohol, drugs, neurotoxic additives, and twisting of the umbilical cord.

- The considerable amount of methanol and phenylalanine in aspartame is relevant (Chapter 9). For example, phenylalanine has the highest affinity for transport across the blood-brain barrier of all circulating amino acids.

- Studies of pregnant diabetics indicate the adverse effects of prenatal metabolic changes—especially increased ketones caused by prolonged fasting—on intelligence (Rizzo 1991).

- In studies of identical twins, neurologic changes tend to occur in the twin suffering decreased oxygen when the umbilical cord became wrapped around its neck.

VERY-LOW-BIRTH WEIGHT AND PREMATURITY

Very-low-birth weight infants with subnormal head circumference at eight months of age tend to have impaired cognitive function and poor academic achievement (Hack 1991).

The neural development of preterm infants who fail to receive enough maternal milk can be markedly impaired because human milk contains long-chain lipids, numerous hormones and other trophic factors essential for brain growth and maturation. This is subsequently evidenced by a low intelligent quotient (IQ) (Lucas 1992).

HEAD TRAUMA

A severe blow to the head, either during a single event or on a repetitive basis, could trigger the pathologic responses found in AD, perhaps by stimulating amyloid precursor protein (APP) (Chapter 4).

- The association of dementia with repeated head trauma is classically illustrated by "dementia pugilistica" among boxers (Hoffman 1991).
- Roberts et al (1991) demonstrated deposition of beta-amyloid in the brains of six patients who survived 6-18 days after suffering a single injury to the head.

Jaret, Mandell and Avitable (1993) emphasized that the term "mild" can be deceptive when applied to head trauma. They analyzed 75 consecutive adults with loss of consciousness or amnesia after non-penetrating head trauma; all had CT scans of the head. Some patients with Glasgow coma scales of 13-14 evidenced internal injuries, possibly requiring neurosurgical intervention.

SEVERE CALORIC RESTRICTION

Severe restriction of calories, whether from voluntary dieting or famine, probably represents a major risk factor for AD. The brain's vulnerability to severe depletion of energy, especially during infancy and childhood, was stressed above and in Chapters 7 and 8.

Attention also is directed to the frequency and severity of arbitrary caloric restriction by women of all ages (Roberts 1985, 1992b). In fact, *National Center for Health Statistics indicate that half the women in the United States are dieting at any given time!* This matter assumes added significance in view of the apparent greater vulnerability of females to AD (see below).

PRIOR SURGERY

Prolonged and repeated surgery, another phenomenon of the 20th Century, probably poses a greater risk for AD than previously envisioned due to the following influences:

- Severe and prolonged lack of oxygen (*The Lancet* 1992; 340:580-582)

- The neurotoxicity of many anesthetic agents and drugs administered before, during and after surgery (Chapter 11)

- Prolonged hypoglycemia during and after surgery resulting from failure to provide adequate nutrition intravenously or by month (Chapter 8)

The dramatic swelling of the brain in the first hour after coronary artery bypass surgery provides a dramatic indication of such postoperative changes. Harris et al (1993) reported this finding by MRI testing immediately after the operation in six patients undergoing "routine" bypass surgery. Various mechanisms could account for them and the stroke or permanent neurophysiological defects noted among such patients—including decreased perfusion of the brain and embolism by air, platelets and fat.

FEMININITY

There is the distinct impression that (1) more women are afflicted with AD, (2) the disease occurs earlier in women than in men, and (3) certain changes of the AD brain are more prominent in women. Indeed, careful epidemiologic studies, corrected for an increased proportion of older women in the at-risk population, appear to have established the fact that femininity is an *independent* risk factor for AD (Blass 1993). (Some disagree.)

- After adjusting for age, females were the preponderant gender in 14 population surveys of AD patients (Henderson 1990).

- A prevalence study of medically-diagnosed dementia patients from the Rochester (Minnesota) population revealed 208 women and 81 men (Kokmen 1989).

- A collaborative study of 1980-1990 prevalence estimates in Europe (Rocca 1991) indicated a higher incidence of AD among women than men in some populations.

- A Framingham study convincingly demonstrated the greater prevalence of dementia among women—i.e., 48.2/1,000 for women, and 30.5/1,000 for men in the biennial Exam 17 cohort of 1982/1983 (Bachman 1992).

- Buckwalter et al (1993) analyzed gender-associated neuropathological features in 70 consecutively autopsied patients with confirmed AD. Women had a significantly greater amount of vascular amyloid.

This apparent gender preponderance is consistent with observations mentioned earlier.

- Reactive hypoglycemia and diabetogenic hyperinsulinism are intensified by female hormones (Chapter 8).

- The use of female hormones increases insulin production and release (Chapter 8).

- Six percent of women between the ages of 45 and 50 currently take contraceptive hormones ("the pill") (Winslow 1991).

- A 3:1 ratio of females to males has been consistently encountered among individuals who developed severe confusion and memory loss after ingesting aspartame products (Chapter 9).

- The problem of severe caloric restriction, chiefly by weight-conscious women, was noted above.

- Aging is associated with a significant rise of large neutral amino acids—especially phenylalanine (Chapter 9)—in the plasma of apparently healthy elderly women, but not men (Caballero 1991).

- Physical and emotional overload has been experienced by "liberated" women during the second half of the 20th Century. This issue is discussed in Chapters 13 and 19.

- The association of apolipoprotein E type 4 with AD (Chapter 3) is more pronounced in women (Poirier 1993).

There is also suggestive evidence that decreased or lost estrogen activity, whether spontaneous or postoperative, can interfere with cognition and memory. This presumably reflects decreased neuronal function and the degeneration of specific neurons from reduced estrogen-sensitive neurotrophins that are necessary for their maintenance, especially basal forebrain cholinergic neurons. Singh and Simpkins (1993) found (1) consistently higher affinity of choline uptake in the frontal cortex and hippocampus in ovariectomized rats, and (2) improvement of impaired learning following ovariectomy with estrogen replacement.

The important role of estrogen in maintaining brain connections, in part by stimulating the choline acetyltransferase required to synthesize acetylcholine (Chapter 5), clarifies several clinical observations (Angier 1994). They include the greater frequency of AD in postmenopausal women, the greater risk for AD among extremely thin women (since estrogen is stored in body fat), and the apparent protection against this disease by hormonal replacement. (It is noteworthy that much of a male's circulating testosterone is converted to estrogen in the brain.)

> This issue remains controversial. Barrett-Connor and Kritz-Silverstein (1993) could not find compelling or consistent evidence that the use of estrogen by older women preserves cognitive function. This inference was based on the direct action of estrogen on choline acetyltransferase (the enzyme synthesizing acetylcholine) (Chapter 5), and altered nerve growth factor physiology in sterilized animal models.

PROLONGED SLEEP DEPRIVATION

Recurrent deprivation of sufficient sleep represents a severe insult to brain function. It commonly results from the combination of long hours at work (including holding multiple jobs), the use of stimulants (e.g., caffeine; illegal drugs), and failure to take rest periods. The habitual "siesta" taken in many countries seems wise in this context.

The importance of sleep deprivation in lowering immune function, especially relative to increased susceptibility to infection, has been shown by multiple observers (Blakeslee 1993). Many concomitant changes could also alter brain function.

> Cytokines normally released by the brain during sleep induce a special firing pattern among diverse neuronal groups that tends to preserve their connections. It may be disrupted by sleep deprivation.

LEFT-HANDEDNESS

Left-handedness (sinistrality) has been reported as being disproportionately more frequent among AD patients (Li 1992, Seltzer 1983). Halpern and Coren (1991) suggested that it might indicate covert neuropathology relating to prenatal-perinatal complications and immune system dysfunction.

Coren (1990) also correlated the combination of advanced maternal age (40 years and older) (see above) and left-handedness in the offspring. The increase of left-handedness—more than twice that found in younger counterparts—was attributed to prenatal and perinatal stress.

HEIGHT

The issue of increased height indirectly invokes the factors of altered nutrition and hyperinsulinism during childhood. Hypoglycemia is a major stimulus to the release of growth hormone (Chapter 8).

EDUCATIONAL ATTAINMENT

The significance of prior formal education and academic achievement, relative to vulnerability to AD, is still debated. In my personal experience, AD has occurred with disturbing frequency among highly educated persons of both genders, albeit possibly in a delayed manner.

A number of studies seem to validate low educational and occupational attainment as risk factors for dementia (Stern 1993, Kokmen 1993, Kahana 1993). Some hold the view that scholastic attainment tends to delay AD because of "increased brain reserve capacity."

- Martinez-Lage et al (1992) concluded that little education and a positive family history of AD were the only definable risk factors in a case-control study of elderly persons in Pamplona (Spain).

- A trend for impaired mental functioning was noted among older persons with low education, compared to others with a high school or post-secondary education (Forbes 1992).

- Kahana et al (1993) emphasized the apparent protective effect of education, relative to senile dementia, in an epidemiologic study of the total population of elderly persons in Ashkelon (Israel). Moreover, the influence of poor education was comparable in both genders, and among Sephardi and Ashkenazi Jews.

- Stern et al (1994) provided additional data suggesting that increased educational and occupational attainment may reduce the risk of AD—either by decreasing the "ease of clinical detection" or by imparting sufficient reserve to delay the onset of its clinical manifestations. The same also applies to certain leisure activities that require intellectual stimulation.

- MRI studies have been used in an attempt to clarify such associations. Reporting a positive correlation between IQ and brain size, Willerman (1991) observed: "Our lower-IQ 20-year-olds have brains that look like those of older people."

Mortimer and Graves (1993) reviewed the strong association between a lower education level and the risk of AD. The mechanisms for such increased risk could reflect (1) reduced "brain reserve capacity" stemming from fetal or early-life exposures associated with lower family socioeconomic status, and (2) the inhibition of neuronal growth resulting from suboptimal lifelong mental stimulation.

There is evidence that dendrites continue to grow even during old age (Buell 1979). This phenomenon was inferred in a study of the cognitive function of 247 Roman Catholic nuns who shared a similar lifestyle, but differed in their educational achievement (Snowdon 1989). The more highly educated were almost twice as likely to survive to ages 75 to 100 years with intact cognitive function, compared to the less educated nuns.

Studies on several animal species confirm that mental stimulation through various mechanisms causes larger nerve cells within the brain and more dendrites (interconnecting projections) from these cells. For example, complex environments tend to stimulate dendritic growth and increase brain weight throughout the life span of animals (Greenough 1981). These findings reinforce the observation that persons with more education who conducted active social and intellectual lives have longer dendrites in the brain at autopsy.

Several other aspects concerning the issue of education as a significant variable in AD should be considered.

- There may be pitfalls when highly educated persons are given tests of "intelligence" and cognitive function.

- Malnutrition and limited schooling due to poverty during childhood could have resulted in suboptimum brain function (Chapter 7).

THE ISSUE OF "AFFLUENCE"

The relatively affluent background of some AD patients should be addressed because it is relevant to many of the risk factors described in previous chapters. Such individuals may have had greater exposure to these adverse influences:

- Increased intake of calories, sugar and protein (Chapter 7)

- Greater consumption of foods exposed to high temperatures during their processing or preparation (Chapter 7)

- The use of potentially neurotoxic additives (Chapter 9) and exotic foods

- Resort to costly drugs for nervous tension, insomnia and weight reduction (Chapter 11)

- More elective surgery requiring anesthesia (Chapter 11)

- Increased air travel—with the associated risk of prolonged hypoxemia and carbon monoxide exposure, especially in newer large aircraft (Chapter 12)

- Extensive dental work entailing anesthesia (local or general) and more amalgam (mercury) fillings (Chapter 11)

- Excessive smoking (see below), drinking, and the use of psychotropic drugs for combatting the considerable stress spawned by business and professional activities (Chapters 13 and 19)

MOBILITY

The suggested influence of considerable mobility on vulnerability to AD relates in part to the associated stress (Chapter 19).

The impression that persons who are more mobile might be at greater risk for AD led to a study by Forbes and McAniey (1992) of 541 participants in the Ontario Longitudinal Study on Aging. They reported an odds ratio of 1.47 for symptoms of impaired mental functioning by persons who had moved more than twice since 1958, compared to 1.00 for infrequent movers.

OTHER POSSIBLE ENVIRONMENTAL INFLUENCES

I. Smoking

The incidence of AD appears to be increased by heavy smoking—perhaps as much as fourfold for one-pack-a-day smokers (Shalat 1989). The contributory effects include exposure to carbon monoxide (Chapter 11) and "tobacco hypoglycemia" (Chapter 8).

This issue remains controversial, however. A reduced risk was reported in one population-based case-controlled study (Brenner 1992). The investigators suggested that the action of nicotine on nicotinic brain receptors causes a release of more acetylcholine (Chapter 5).

> Riggs (1993) cautioned that the differential survival between smokers and non-smokers could result in gene pools—including variable DNA repair mechanisms—sufficiently different to account for the negative association (apparent neuroprotection) between AD and smoking.

II. Prior Occupational Exposures

Exposure to many environmental neurotoxins at work (Chapter 11) could be conducive to subsequent AD.

Dartigues et al (1991) found that poor memory performance for both visual recognition and verbal-induced recall correlated strongly with prior lifetime occupation. This epidemiologic study involved nondemented elderly residents in the Bordeaux area of France. The risk for poor memory performance was as much as three times higher among farmers, domestic service employees, and blue-collar workers than professionals and managers. Furthermore, it was independent of educational attainment and familiarity with the testing situation.

III. The Adverse Effects of Artificial Light

This risk factor remains controversial. It is appropriately introduced by referring again to the fact that AD has emerged as a phenomenon of the 20th Century (Introduction to Section I).

The adverse effects of artificial lighting deserve consideration in view of the following facts:

- Tungsten filament lamps did not become available commercially until the early 1900s.

- Exposure to lighting is ubiquitous. Persons in the United States commonly spend 90 percent of their time indoors.

- Ordinary incandescent light has little ultraviolet, and is deficient in the blue end of the spectrum.

- "Natural white" fluorescent lighting also differs from the full spectrum of natural sunlight.

The relevant details include the physiological effects of light and the metabolism of melatonin ("the hormone of darkness"). John N. Ott (1973), a pioneer in this field, aptly likened "malillumination" to malnutrition. As a case in point, the high red content within the spectrum of incandescent light bulbs causes profound changes in both plant and animal cell walls.

Another important orientation concerns the extraordinary impact on both the timing system ("body clock") and sleep patterns resulting from artificial lighting, combined with contemporary habits of living and working. For example, persons having a form of insomnia associated with insufficient sleep and chronic fatigue, referred to as the delayed sleep phase syndrome (DSPS), prefer to sleep at hours not compatible with conventional life cycles.

The following observations underscore the potential adverse influences of artificial lighting.

- There is considerable evidence that chronic "light shock" or "radiation stress" can profoundly alter brain function. Such stress encompasses sudden exposure to lighting in darkness, abnormal spectra of artificial lighting (especially from fluorescent fixtures), defective light bulbs and fixtures, and "visual pollution" from extended viewing of movies, television and video terminals.

- Artificial light behind window glass and in buildings without windows markedly distorts the wave-length energy entering the eyes, compared to natural sunlight.

- Repeated exposure to long-wave ultraviolet light from artificial sources, and a lack or deficiency of exposure to sunlight, could interfere with important immunologic mechanisms (Hersey 1983, Fuller 1992).

- Exposure to fluorescent light seems more strongly linked to melanoma than to education or social class (Beral 1982).

IV. Prolonged Wearing of Sunglasses

The habitual wearing of sunglasses introduces considerations similar to those mentioned above. Dark sunglasses tend to filter out more of the ultraviolet and some other shorter wave lengths of sunlight energy. Furthermore, glass color can alter the characteristics of light.

V. Other Sources of Radiation Stress

Repeated exposure to significant <u>electromagnetic radiation,</u> another technologic achievement of the 20th Century, influences brain function… probably in a cumulative manner. Ott (1973) summarized the prior literature indicating changes in acetylcholine (Chapter 5) after exposure to ultra high frequency (UHF) radio fields. There is evidence that electromagnetic fields increase the number of calcium ions within nerve cells grown in the laboratory, which in turn can be neurotoxic.

Most persons in our society live in a field of "electromagnetic chaos." This refers to random and disordered photons that can pass through nearly everything—including lead. The effects on radio signals when driving under high tension power lines provide a well-known instance.

There are many sources of such radiation. They include <u>television</u> (see below), <u>microwave ovens, long distance telephone microwave relay towers, x-ray machines, diathermy, radio and television broadcasting stations, office machines</u> (including copiers, fax machines and some types of computers), <u>radar devices</u> (e.g., units carried by police officers to detect and document speeding), <u>electric blankets, electric hair dryers, dish-washers, electrically operated alarms, industrial and home sewing machines</u> (see below) and a new generation of <u>mobile cellular phones</u> with frequencies above 100,000 Herz.

- Impairment of short-term memory has been reported with exposure to 60 Hz.

- Microwaving also can convert L-form amino acids (such as proline) to potentially neurotoxic D-forms.

- The levels for electric shavers range from 14-1600 milligauss (mG), and for hair dryers from 3-14 mG. (The standard for safety of electromagnetic radiation proposed by the EPA is one mG.)

Dr. Eugene Sobel reported to the 1994 Fourth International Conference on Alzheimer's Disease and Related Disorders that persons with a high occupational exposure to electromagnetic fields are at least three times as likely to develop AD as those without significant exposure. Dressmakers and tailors were found to be over-represented among AD victims.

The impact on brain development of the fetus when pregnant women are exposed to <u>video display terminals,</u> in terms of subsequent neurodegeneration, has yet to be evaluated. (More than 20 million working women in the United States currently utilize this equipment.) There is a basis for such concern.

> A study in Finland indicated a triple rate of miscarriage for clerical workers (at three different firms) exposed to high levels of an extremely low frequency (ELF) electromagnetic field (*The Miami Herald* December 9, 1992, p. A-9).

VI. <u>Prolonged Television Viewing in Childhood</u>

Habitual watching of television during the first decade has become a tragedy of human development in our society. It will have to be taken more seriously as a major risk factor for AD among recent generations exposed to such "entertainment."

This admonition involves more than the issue of radiation stress (see above). Exposure to such passive pseudoimagery during the first seven years prevents the brain from developing many pathways vital for proper "internal metaphoric imagery."

Educators now realize that memory, learning, intellectual creativity, and even immunity are optimized by natural "linguistic intelligence." It derives from reading and story-telling by parents, frequent discussions involving the entire family, conventional play with siblings and friends, and listening to radio or cassettes aimed at stimulating the imagination of young listeners.

The toll of excessive television viewing has been increased by concomitant adverse social and neurotoxic phenomena that deprive young children of legitimate models and a wholesome nurturing environment. They include erosion of the nuclear and extended family (creating a vacuum for television to serve as a surrogate babysitter), excessive intellectual demands made too early in life, and the dumping of toxic chemicals and drugs (e.g., estrogens and growth hormones in water and food) onto the home nest (Chapter 10 and 11).

There is comparable concern about children and teenagers who become immersed in impersonal computer networks. They also risk becoming electronic hermits in this "new kind of public space."

"MENTAL DECLINE IN OLD AGE": FURTHER INSIGHTS

Several researchers have emphasized that high mental functioning can be maintained in old age, albeit with wide variations based on various factors (Coleman 1994).

- Men tend to preserve spatial orientation, as illustrated by the ability to read a map correctly or to assemble a piece of furniture from printed directions.

- Women appear more likely to maintain inductive reasoning, as in assessing the information in a bus timetable.

A number of influences favor the retention of mental function. They include a flexible attitude, continued physical activity, good lung function that minimizes hypoxia (Chapter 12), a prior successful career, and active involvement and continued keen interests after retirement.

The importance of living with a high-functioning spouse should be acknowledged. The cognitive value of such a relationship explains in part the dramatic deterioration of some persons after such a spouse becomes ill or dies.

SECTION IV

MEASURES THAT MAY PREVENT, MINIMIZE OR DELAY THE ONSET OF ALZHEIMER'S DISEASE

*Old age is like any thing else. You've got
to start early to be good at it.*

Fred Astaire

*I am an out-and-out believer in preventive measures against
diseases, as contrasted with what are curative agencies.*

Dr. Oliver Wendell Holmes (1892)

*Surely, if a safe and effective preventive therapy is available to shift the
earlier distribution curves later, the concerns of individuals will be
reduced. We are all at risk of developing scurvy, yet vitamin C
prevents the disease. Vitamin C is safe and effective, and no one
is concerned about the genetic risk of scurvy.**

A. D. Roses et al (1994)

*Population morbidity from Alzheimer disease may be substantially
reduced if new strategies succeed in identifying those who are
predisposed to it and in delaying an otherwise unavoidable onset by
some years. In the example given, the morbidity from Alzheimer
disease could be reduced by half if onset were delayed by only
5 years. Attempts to postpone onset by pharmacologic intervention or by manipulation of the environment offer hope
of substantial prevention of morbidity in Alzheimer disease.***

Dr. John C.S. Breitner (1991)

This section offers a <u>rational</u> program aimed at preventing, minimizing or delaying the onset of Alzheimer's disease (AD). Defense Against Alzheimer's Disease (DAAD®) is largely based on (1) the concept of a "transitional" phase that probably averages 30 years (Beyruther 1991), and (2) likely risk factors, reviewed in previous chapters, which can be constructively addressed.

Nerves cells that are lost because of disease or the effects of neurotoxins cannot be replaced. Many of the remaining ones, however, retain a remarkable capacity for healing. The full extent of such repair has been appreciated only recently (Jenkins 1991). Breitner (1991) projected *that the current morbidity from AD could be reduced 50 percent by postponing its clinical onset for five years.* Additionally, the preservation of cognitive function appears to favor longer survival (Perls 1992).

Such a program must be approached in the light of these caveats and disclaimers:

- DAAD is a long-term commitment. Yet, its merit should appeal to intelligent individuals concerned about becoming victims of the unrelenting AD epidemic.

- There is no guarantee that AD or another degenerative brain disorder will not develop in persons who follow this type of regimen.

- Doubtless, the program will require modification as additional insights evolve, and as new therapies (not necessarily drugs) become available.

- "Healing" of selective neurons is not synonymous with "curing" AD. This distinction accounts for my emphasis on both the delay of AD and maintaining one's "vital" or "working" memory.

- The advice of a physician should be sought whenever any suggestion herein differs from a professional recommendation. For instance, my controversial reservations about avoiding products that contain aspartame (NutraSweet®), monosodium glutamate (MSG), aluminum antacids, fluoridated water, and megadoses of vitamin E reflect published observations made over many years of medical practice.

Persons with major risk factors must recognize that NOW is the best time to embark upon such a program for influencing their future health. (Some wise soul said, "The best way of predicting the future is to shape it.") This theme also might be phrased "New ideas to prevent old brains" or "Saging instead of aging."

This type of responsible program is based on much factual material, and ought to be welcomed for several reasons. They include the gruesome epidemiologic statistics (Chapter 2), the relative ineffectiveness of drug therapy in reversing dementia of the Alzheimer type, the focus on enlightened hygiene, and the need for ongoing awareness and vigilance about reducing exposure to many neurotoxic chemicals present in the air, water, food and consumer goods.

> The recurring emphasis on "do not" measures may be disconcerning to some readers who primarily seek "do" listings. Advice about abstinence in human behavior given by sages of earlier generations provides important precedents. The *Sefer Ha-Mitzvoth* (Book of Worthy Deeds) was written by Maimonides between the years 1168-1170. At that time, he functioned as both an eminent physician and leader of the Egyptian Jewish community. Maimonides asserted that observation of 613 commandments—248 "positive" and 365 "negative"—enabled man to lead a life of harmony and happiness consonant with God's divine will.

I do not expect some "magic bullet" capable of reversing "early" AD, notwithstanding repeated glowing preliminary reports by corporate-funded researchers. (I hope to be proved wrong.) In this regard, Megalli and Friedman (1991) emphasized the need for skepticism about information under the guise of impartial educational material from allegedly neutral or independent sources that prove to be corporate front groups.

- A century ago, Oliver Wendell Holmes (1892) properly emphasized hygiene and "simple living" over "potent potions of the pharmacy" to prevent disease.

- Growdon (1992) summarized the disappointing results of many attempts at palliative drug treatment in this commentary:

  "Pending discovery of another neurotransmitter deficit that fully accounts for the dementia, it is now time to abandon simple replacement therapy and to develop treatments that can affect the fundamental mechanisms of neuronal degeneration. Future attempts to treat the disorder will follow strategies to restore neuronal function, protect neuronal survival, or prevent neurons from dying in the first place."*

The ability to prevent or delay this disease through conscious effort raises centuries-old philosophic issues. Some deal with the controversy over the ability of man's free will to direct his destiny regardless of whether neural predestination is governed by genetics or the laws of chemistry and physics. Both authors of the Old Testament and Saint Augustine contended that God had given man the gift of free will with which to follow the good impulse (*yetzer ha-tov*). The related arguments by Spinoza in the 17th Century are equally germane.

---

*©1992 *New England Journal of Medicine.* Reproduced with permission.

17

AVOIDANCE AND CONTROL OF RISK FACTORS:
A SYSTEM ANALYSIS APPROACH

*As to diseases, make a habit of two things—to help,
or at least to do no harm.*

Hippocrates (*Epidemics*)

*The proper use of hypothesis is the mark of the good practicing
physician, the good research physician, and the good medical
teacher. All of them recognize that a good hypothesis
must bring together scattered data.*

M. D. Altschule (1966)

*We owe our children a set of good habits; for habit is to be either
their best friend or their worst enemy, not only during
childhood, but through all the years.*

George Herbert Betts (1868-1934)

The following listings are a condensation of reasonable precautionary measures and prudent advice aimed at preventing, minimizing or delaying Alzheimer's disease (AD). Their rationale is indicated by references to previous chapters wherein the topic was considered. When appropriate, some measures appear under several categories.

Admittedly, no individual can indefinitely follow every recommendation for a variety of reasons—personal, economic, technologic and political. A constant awareness of them, however, is likely to effect beneficial changes involving behavior, preferences and life style. Special emphasis is placed on pregnancy and child-rearing.

158

PRECAUTIONARY MEASURES TO BE TAKEN BY WOMEN OF CHILD-BEARING AGE, ESPECIALLY DURING PREGNANCY
(Chapters 7 and 18)

- Avoid severe physical fatigue (e.g., exhausting exercise)
- Avoid smoking
- Avoid poor nutrition
- Avoid prolonged fasting
- Avoid dehydration by drinking at least six glasses of water daily
- Avoid overeating
- Avoid excessive sugar and highly sweetened foods
- Avoid alcohol if pregnant or attempting to become pregnant (see below)
- Avoid fish that appears to be spoiled (improper storage or refrigeration) or suspected of contamination

    Polychlorinated biphenyls (PCBs) present in swordfish, salmon, tuna

    Impaired cognitive development can result from prenatal exposure (Chen 1992)

    Fish from water known to be high in mercury

    Hepatitis virus in clams from raw sewage in endemic areas

- Avoid fish that might cause ciguatera poisoning, especially during pregnancy (Chapter 18)

    In the Southeast, they include large grouper, red snapper and barracuda

    Yellowtail snapper and mahimahi are generally not problems

- Avoid food and beverage products containing aspartame (NutraSweet®; Equal®) (Chapters 9 and 18)
- Avoid monosodium glutamate (manufactured glutamic acid; MSG) and related compounds, such as hydrolyzed vegetable protein (HVP) (Chapters 9 and 18)

    This does not refer to glutamic acid or glutamate present in unadulterated protein

- Avoid excessive iron (Chapters 9 and 18)

    Including numerous "fortified" cereals and nutritional supplements containing iron

    A pregnant woman who does not need iron for an iron-deficiency anemia should avoid such supplementation

- Avoid ALL drugs—both by prescription and over-the-counter (see below)

    If attempting to become pregnant, discuss their need and side effects with a doctor

- Avoid or minimize pesticide residues in food (Chapter 11)

    Wash and peel fruits and vegetables

If appropriate, use a vegetable scrub brush; add a few drops of mild soap (without perfume or dyes) while washing them

Squeeze some lemon juice in the water when washing leafy vegetables, but leave the greens in no longer than one minute

If buying fresh "organic" food, request proof of third-party certification

Minor imperfections do not affect flavor or quality

Buy foods in season to avoid produce imported from countries having less strict pesticide regulations

- Avoid exposure to environmental pesticides (Chapter 11)
- Avoid other potentially toxic substances in the environment, including the following:

Fluoridated water and fluoride-containing toothpaste (Chapter 11) (see below)

Polychlorinated biphenyls (PCBs)

Water and air possibly contaminated by arsenic from nearby smelting plants and toxic dumps (Chapter 11)

- Avoid food stored in ceramic dishware that may contain lead (see below)
- Avoid or minimize radiation exposure—both diagnostic and environmental

Including prolonged television viewing (Chapter 16), and video display terminals (VDTs) because available VDT screens do not block the emitted radiation

- Avoid toxic chemicals and other hazards in the workplace or with hobbies (Chapter 11)
- Avoid prolonged and excessive air travel, especially in newer large aircraft (Chapter 12)

Reflects the possible risk of decreased oxygen availability, and increased exposure to carbon monoxide (Tolchin 1993)

PRECAUTIONARY MEASURES TO BE TAKEN WITH INFANTS AND CHILDREN

- Insist upon measures aimed at avoiding severe hypoglycemia (Chapter 8)

Especially in the newborn

- Encourage breast-feeding (Chapter 18), and drinking at least six glasses of water daily
- Avoid arbitrary bottle-feeding of formulas based on modified cow's milk (Chapters 7 and 18)

Especially in the case of pre-term infants

Immune responses to cow's-milk albumin causing pancreatic islet-cell dysfunction can result in diabetes (Karjalainen 1992)

- Routinely feed infants during the night

If feeding formula is used, do not overheat it (Chapters 7 and 18)

- Avoid the unnecessary intake of lead (Chapter 11), aluminum (Chapter 10), fluoride (Chapter 11), and arsenic (Chapter 11) in infant feeding formulas through the precautions described below

    E.g., do not use hot tap water for baby formula because it risks the introduction of lead

- Limit the amount of fruit juices given infants and young children

    Large quantities, especially apple juice, can cause diarrhea and hinder development (Webb 1994)

- Resist buying the avalanche of new products aimed at child consumers that contain excessive sugar and artifical colorings

    This alarming trend is conducive both to obesity and a variety of neuropsychiatric problems

- Avoid giving infants the following:

    Aluminum-containing antacids (Chapter 10)

    Excessive iron (Chapters 9 and 18)—the feeding of infants with pasteurized milk and baby formulas containing synthetic iron is increasingly challenged

    Products containing aspartame and manufactured glutamic acid (MSG) (Chapters 9 and 18)

- Parents and teachers should check that materials used in arts and crafts by children have appropriate safety testing and labeling

    Crayons and chalk from the Far East may contain lead

    Such labeling includes "AP NONTOXIC," "CP NONTOXIC," and "HEALTH LABEL"

    Other precautions entail avoidance of putting any materials in the mouth, the wearing of smocks, and the prohibition of eating or drinking in the work area

- Avoid exposure to cigarette smoke ("passive smoking") (Chapter 12)

- Insist upon the adequate immunization of children

    Can prevent the encephalitis complicating bacterial and viral "childhood" infections

EMPHASIZE PROPER NUTRITION, EATING HABITS AND OTHER HYGIENIC MEASURES DURING THE CHILDHOOD YEARS (Chapters 7 and 18) BY TEACHING CHILDREN TO:

- Eat slowly

- Chew food well

- Avoid missing meals

    Especially girls who "fear fat" (Chapter 18)

- Minimize the intake of sugar and highly sweetened foods (Chapters 7 and 18)
- Take sugar-free snacks during the midafternoon and at bedtime
- Avoid excessively heated meat, fish and milk (Chapter 7 and 18)
- Avoid municipally fluoridated water (Chapter 11)

    Fluoride cannot be removed by a carbon filter
- Avoid products containing aspartame (NutraSweet®) (Chapters 9 and 18)
- Avoid manufactured monosodium glutamate (MSG) and related substances (Chapters 9 and 18)
- Avoid other suspected neurotoxic additives (Chapter 9)
- Avoid or minimize radiation exposure

    Both diagnostic and environmental—including prolonged television viewing
- Avoid recently-marketed novel foods that may not have been adequately tested in humans
- Avoid exposure to excessive aluminum (see below)
- Avoid utensils, old pewter, ceramic, decaled or lead-crystal cups that may contain lead (Chapter 11)
- Avoid excessive iron (Chapters 7, 11 and 8)

    Including "fortified" cereals and supplements containing iron
- Avoid "passive" smoking from adults who smoke

EMPHASIZE INTELLECTUAL STIMULATION AND THE ADEQUATE EDUCATION OF CHILDREN

General Considerations

   *Low educational achievement appears to be a significant risk factor for AD (Chapter 16)
   *Numerous clinical and experimental observations underscore the importance of providing infants and children with adequate sensory input and experiences in order to influence brain development
   *Failure to do so can negatively impact the brain through failure to stimulate the connections between cells known as synapses
   *Providing young children with quantity time through reading to them, encouraging music lessons, and other interactions can have lifelong cognitive benefits
   *Society ought to encourage the process by expanding family leave (e.g., to six months) and expanding the Head Start program to children below the age of three

- Emphasize reading and story-telling by parents, frequent discussions with the entire family, and play by siblings in the early years to develop "linguistic intelligence"

    Such natural models and innate intellectual nurturing stimulate numerous path ways within the brain that serve to enhance memory, learning and creativity

- Discourage prolonged television viewing (Chapter 16)

- Encourage formal education and extracurricular activities (especially music and the arts) to the highest practical and available level

    Example: listening to Mozart's piano music for 10 minutes significantly improved performance in intelligence tests taken thereafter (even among university students who did not like it) —presumably by stimulating neural pathways important to cognition (*The New York Times* October 14, 1993, p. B-1).

PROPER NUTRITIONAL HABITS BY ADULTS

(Chapters 7, 8 and 18)

General Considerations

    *Carefully read labels on food and beverage products
    *Be suspicious of all "new and improved" or "novelty" foods, and the additives contained therein—as well as the original products being "improved"

- Avoid the severe restriction of calories and arbitrary fasting for reasons of vanity, especially fast-weight-loss programs without professional supervision

    Caloric restriction should be avoided by nonobese women having an inappropriate fear of obesity (Chapters 16 and 18)

- Learn the habit of eating slowly and savoring food by chewing it thoroughly

    Rapid eating can create a "dumping effect," and thereby precipitate hypoglycemia ("low blood sugar attacks") (Chapter 8)

- Utilize the technique of "scientific nibbling" (snacks) if prone to hypoglycemia

- Avoid excessive amounts of sugar and highly sweetened foods (Chapters 7 and 8)

- Drink at least six glasses of water daily unless medically contraindicated
    Hydration assists brain metabolism and the elimination of metallic and other neurotoxins

- Select citrus fruits rather than citrus juices

- Avoid excessive amounts of foods with concentrated natural sugars
    E.g., raisins; prunes; apricots; figs; mangos; dates

- Avoid excessive decaffeinated coffee
    Ground Swiss water-processed decaffeinated beans are preferable

- Avoid products containing aspartame (NutraSweet®) (Chapters 9 and 18)
    Over 5,000 products are presently sweetened with it

- Avoid manufactured monosodium glutamate (MSG) and related neurotoxic additives (Chapters 9 and 18)

    Be aware of misleading labels—including hydrolyzed vegetable protein (HVP); "sodium caseinate"; "autolyzed yeast"

- Avoid foods subjected to very high temperatures (Chapters 7 and 18)

    Uncommon D-stereoisomers of amino acids are increased in charred, heavily roasted or barbecued meat, poultry, and smoked fish

- Check or avoid drinking water from wells in the vicinity of toxic dump sites, smelting plants and coal burning industries—especially for arsenic contamination (Chapter 11)

- Avoid the use of aluminum pots and pans
- Avoid beverages in aluminum cans (see below)
- Avoid common foods that may be causing sensitivity reactions (Chapter 18)

    The common sensitizers include corn (also corn starch and oils), wheat, milk, eggs, peanuts, soybeans

    If tolerated to some degree, rotate them, and avoid their frequent consumption

- Avoid any processed foods suspected of causing adverse reactions (Chapter 18) due to:

    Certain artificial colors (such as tartrazine)

    Preservatives (such as sulfiting agents)

    Ripening procedures (ethylene gas)

    Protective waxes

    Packaging (especially some plastics used in microwaving)

- Limit the use of exotic and highly seasoned "gourmet" foods

    They are apt to be low in nutritional value, and to contain sensitizing agents

- Avoid "guilt-free" new foods that were insufficiently tested for safety (Chapters 9 and 11)

    Minimize those with controversial additives (e.g., aspartame), even when designated Generally Recognized As Safe (GRAS)

- Avoid adding excessive lactase (Lactaid®) to milk

    Increases the absorption of galactose, a potential neurotoxin at high levels (Chapter 9)

- Avoid or minimize pesticide residues in food (Chapter 11)

    Insecticides, pesticides and other chemicals can be removed or reduced from vegetables and fruits by washing or bathing in vinegar, a detergent, or hydrogen peroxide (one quarter cup in a sink full of cold water)

    Wash and peel fruits and vegetables

        Use a vegetable scrub brush, if appropriate

        Add a few drops of mild soap (without perfume or dyes) while washing them

        Squeeze some lemon juice in the water when washing leafy vegetables, but leave the greens in no longer than one minute

    If buying fresh "organic" food, request proof of third-party certification

        Minor imperfections do not affect flavor or quality

        Buy foods in season to avoid produce imported from countries having less strict pesticide regulations

GENERAL PRECAUTIONARY MEASURES FOR ADULTS

• Avoid *excessive* reduction of blood pressure from over- aggressive treatment of hypertension (see below)

> Small strokes may occur, especially in "border zones" of the brain (Binswanger's disease)

• Take precautions to avoid severe lung disease that can result in reduced oxygen intake (Chapter 12)

> Avoid cigarette smoke—both active and passive

> Obtain adequate treatment for severe bronchitis and pneumonia

> Insist on precautions to minimize occupational lung disorders—e.g., mining; the processing of sugar cane and cotton

> Older persons and high-risk patients (lung disease; heart disease; diabetes) should request Pneumovax® immunization against pneumococcal pneumonia

• Take reasonable precautions to prevent head injury in the event of an automobile accident

> Use three-point and lap restraints

> Prefer vehicles with air bags

• Avoid severe sleep deprivation (Chapter 16)

> Minimize the use of stimulants (e.g., caffeine; amphetamines)

• Take a nap during the day if prone to severe sleepiness (narcolepsy) (Chapter 15)

• Check drinking water for contamination, and institute reasonable precautionary measures

> According to law, consumers must be furnished the results of water tests

> Request a current assay of all substances in "spring" water before purchase

> Test water from a private well for chemicals if it is within several miles of a chemical plant, refinery, land fill, gas station, military base, ranch or farms

> One cannot assume that bottled waters are safer if they represent "bulk" filtered tap water

> Request testing of water when there are odors or persistent stains on laundry or on sinks (particularly for excessive iron, copper, manganese), and if the water is cloudy (turbid)

> Tap water should be run at least 30 seconds whenever it has not been used for several hours

>> Running it to become as cool as possible signifies that it is being drawn from the service pipe outside the house

> If an approved activated carbon filter is used to treat water in the home, the cartridge should be replaced at specified intervals

>> E.g., within a year for a family of four

Distilled water filtered through carbon and ozonated is preferable to spring water, which increasingly tends to be contaminated

Carbon block or other charcoal filters effectively remove chlorine, fluoride and some other particulates, especially in combination with reverse osmosis

Salt-softened water may cause problems

Calcium and magnesium are lost, and replaced with sodium

MINIMIZE INFLUENCES THAT CAN STIMULATE EXCESSIVE INSULIN AND DECREASE BRAIN GLUCOSE DURING HYPOGLYCEMIA ("LOW BLOOD SUGAR ATTACKS") (Chapter 8)

• Avoid arbitrary and extended fasting

• Avoid excessive intake of sugar and highly sweetened foods

• Avoid intensely sweet (sugar) substitutes, even if low in calories

They tend to stimulate the cephalic (brain) phase of insulin secretion and release

• Avoid excessive protein

• Avoid excessive caffeine

• Avoid alcohol or limit its use

Alcohol-induced hypoglycemia can be severe and prolonged

• Avoid smoking ("tobacco hypoglycemia")

• Diabetics should avoid excessive doses of insulin and oral hypoglycemic drugs

Especially long-acting oral agents—e.g., chlorpropamide (Diabinese®)

Along with such medication, snacks MUST be taken in the afternoon, at bedtime, and possibly during the night (especially by persons who retire early)

• Avoid drugs that stimulate excessive insulin and decrease glucose (sugar) tolerance when other options exist

E.g., oral contraceptives; thiazide diuretics

• Avoid excessive and unaccustomed physical exercise

Especially when the tendency to severe reactive hypoglycemia exists (Klachko 1968), and if medication is required for the control of diabetes

AVOID TAKING LARGE AMOUNTS ("MEGADOSES") OF THESE FOLLOWING VITAMINS AND MINERALS UNLESS SPECIFICALLY PRESCRIBED AND MONITORED BY A KNOWLEDGEABLE PROFESSIONAL

General Considerations

*Supplementation with modest amounts of micronutrients might improve the

immune responses associated with aging (Chandra 1992)

Megadoses may impair immunity and possibly lead to dependency states

- Vitamin A (fat-soluble)

- Vitamin B-3 (niacin)

- Vitamin B-6 (pyridoxine)

    Avoid more than 200 mg daily

    Pyridoxine neurotoxicity (based on symptoms, signs, and altered sensory thresholds) has been demonstrated in healthy persons using 1,000-3,000 mg daily (Berger 1992)

    Pyridoxine-dependent epilepsy is a recognized disorder of glutamate metabolism (Chapter 8)

- Vitamin C (ascorbic acid) (see Chapter 18)

    Megadoses can induce a dependency state, with a "rebound" reaction if is withdrawn suddenly

    Avoid taking ascorbic acid and citrate with antacids that contain aluminum hydroxide, especially by patients having chronic kidney disease (Domingo 1991)

- Vitamin D (fat-soluble)

- Vitamin E (fat-soluble) (see Chapter 18) (Roberts 1993)

- Dolomite or bonemeal (taken as sources of calcium)

    Some batches have been contaminated by excessive lead, mercury, arsenic and aluminum (Roberts 1983)

- Fluoride (Chapter 8) (see below)

- Iron (Chapters 8 and 11)

    Alone, or with vitamin-mineral supplements

    Also present in many "fortified" cereals and bakery goods

- Zinc

    Avoid excessive zinc supplements—probably greater than 25-50 mg daily

    High zinc levels outside neurons may turn amyloid into plaque by changing its solubility, and protecting it from enzymatic breakdown (Bush 1994)

MINIMIZE EXPOSURE TO ALUMINUM (Chapter 10) BY AVOIDING OR REDUCING THE FOLLOWING USES:

- Aluminum foil in contact with foods and beverages

- Aluminum cookware and utensils

    Aluminum may increase 75-fold in water when it is heated to 88 degrees C in an aluminum pot (Jackson 1989)

- Aluminum cans

Particularly beer containers

Aluminum content is greater in soft drinks from cans than bottles (Duggan 1992)

• Aluminum-containing antacids—numerous popular products

Tums® contain only calcium carbonate

• Over-the-counter pain relievers buffered with aluminum products

E.g., Ascriptin®; Bufferin®; Vanquish®

• Aluminum-containing baking powders

Aluminum-free ones are available

• Bleached flour in which aluminum is used as a processing aid

• Parmesan and grated cheeses

• Processed cheese in cheeseburgers (aluminum provides the necessary melting quality)

• Various processed foods

E.g., pickles; relishes

• Aluminum-containing antiperspirants and deodorants

• Aluminum-containing douche preparations

E.g., Massengil®; Summer's Eve®

• Fluoridated water (see below)

Fluoride might increase the leaching of aluminum from utensils

Steam distillation of water minimizes aluminum

• Excessive consumption of strong tea

The tea plant *(Camellia sinensis)* concentrates aluminum taken up from acid soil into its leaves

Tea leaves from Darjeeling, Ceylon and Assam tend to have a greater aluminum content

MINIMIZE LEAD EXPOSURES
(Chapter 8)

General considerations

*The brain neurofibrillary tangles found in lead poisoning resemble those seen in AD (Chapter 4)

*Lead is present in most water fixtures

Old pipes and solder release lead

*Some pediatricians recommend testing all children for lead in their blood at the ages of one and two

A high level should initiate search for the source

*Sampling capillary blood in young children to determine lead levels is an acceptable alternative to drawing blood from a vein ((Schlenker 1994)

    If the level is excessive, a confirmatory venous blood lead level should be obtained before intervening with chelation or other therapy

*Request a check of the lead concentration in drinking water from fountains at elementary schools

*Dishware can be tested for lead glaze by pouring vinegar into the vessel, and then adding sodium sulfide

    A black, murky substance will form if lead is present

*Near-total removal of lead from water at home can be obtained by replacing pumps containing lead alloys with pumps made of plastic and stainless steel, or with a reverse osmosis filter

- Take precautions in areas with water that contains excessive lead (above 15 ppb) (Gutfeld 1992), especially in an environment of metal smelters

    Blood lead levels in exposed children should not exceed 0.5 micrograms/liter

    Everywhere, allow the tap water to run for several minutes before drawing it for consumption or food preparation—particularly the first supply in the morning

    If away for a while, let the water run longer to flush out pipes thoroughly

    Avoid excessive boiling of water because the lead concentration tends to increase

    Hot acidic beverages (e.g., coffee) tend to leach lead from glazed ceramic ware, old pewter, and ceramic, decaled or lead-crystal cups

- Do not store food in opened metal cans (as practiced by one-fifth of all households) because the solder may contain lead

- Wash vegetables which may have been grown in lead-containing soil

- Trim the leaves of vegetables

    For example, the outer leaves of cabbage may contain five times more lead than the inner leaves

- Avoid storing alcoholic beverages in lead crystal or ceramic containers (decanters)

- Avoid wine in bottles capped with tin-coated lead capsule
Being replaced by non-leaded caps

- Avoid draft beers served through bronze and brass equipment

- Avoid certain imported ethnic foods that may contain considerable lead

    E.g., Asian pickles; canned okra

- Avoid hair dyes that contain lead
Used both by women and men

- Avoid contact with old paint that may contain lead

    With emphasis upon exposure of children to paint chips, flakes, and dust in pre-1970 houses

- Do not reconstitute infant formulas with lead-contaminated water or lead-contaminated kettles

    Flush the water system with cold water for two minutes before use (see above)

    When in doubt, use bottled water

- Avoid chewing on the plastic insulation of wires (primarily at work)

    Lead compounds are used to color plastics, and as stabilizers in the manufacture of polyvinyl chlorides

MINIMIZE EXCESSIVE FLUORIDE INTAKE

(Chapter 11)

General Considerations

    *Information about the fluoride content of water can be obtained from a local or regional water department

    *Consider the purchase of distilled water or a home water distiller in naturally- or municipally- fluoridated areas

    *Fluoride cannot be removed by a carbon filter without concomitant reverse osmosis

- Avoid or minimize the use of products that contain fluoride

    If a fluoridated toothpaste is used, apply no more than the size of a small pea to the brush, and then rinse mouth thoroughly with water; do not swallow the residue

    Mouthwashes with fluoride

    Dental treatments

        Do not consent to routine topical fluoride applications for children

    Vitamin-mineral preparations with fluoride

        The fluoride is not needed in fluoridated areas

    Commercial soups, soft drinks, juice drinks, beer and wine bottled in fluoridated areas

- Avoid fruit juices made from concentrate prepared in fluoridated areas

    Prefer full-strength 100% pure juices because no water need be added

- Avoid products that tend to contain considerable fluoride

        E.g., cornflakes; some other breakfast cereals

- Avoid fruits, vegetables and grains known to be grown in areas polluted by industrial waste

    Especially the manufacture of aluminum, phosphate, steel, clay and glass

    Fluoride-contaminated phosphate shipped from several areas in Florida is used as a supplement in animal feed and fertilizer, and as a food additive

• Request that fluoride-containing anesthetics be avoided or minimized

> E.g., halothane; enflurane

AVOID OR MINIMIZE ALL DRUGS

(Chapters 9, 11 and 18)

• Restrict the use of <u>prescription drugs</u> as much as possible (see Commentary below)

• Restrict the use of <u>over-the-counter drugs</u> as much as possible (see Commentary below)

> Cold remedies that contain dextromethorphan (e.g., Robitussin DM®) may cause confusion

> Appetite suppressants

• Avoid <u>cocaine and other drugs of abuse</u>

> This is especially important for potential mothers, and men who are attempting to conceive (Yazidi 1991)

• Avoid <u>arbitrary and unnecessary surgery</u>

• Avoid <u>general</u> anesthesia if other options exist

Commentary

If one is concerned about preserving memory, ALL drugs should be avoided or minimized. They include prescription medications, over-the-counter products, "street" drugs, and even such common stimulants as coffee, tea and tobacco. For example, the excessive use of analgesic drugs, such as acetaminophen (Tylenol®), for chronic headache not only can aggravate the condition, but also alters important neurotransmitter mechanisms (e.g., serotonin).

Patients <u>must</u> discuss and clarify the nature of prescribed medications with their physician(s). This precaution is uniquely appropriate when potent tranquilizers and sedatives are taken over prolonged periods for some "functional" disorder—e.g., preparations containing both belladonna and phenobarbital (Donnatal®) for an irritable bowel. When the treatment proves effective, a reduction of dosage may obviate memory problems.

<u>Both</u> physicians and patients should be aware of the potential for interference with memory and intelligence by frequently prescribed drugs. This useful classification is modified after Dr. Thomas D. Sabin (cited by Mark 1992).

• <u>Psychiatric Drugs</u>

> Barbiturates (phenobarbital; Nembutal®; Seconal®)

> Bromides

> Benzodiazepines (Valium®; Librium®)

Phenothiazines (Thorazine®; Prolixin®; Compazine®; Mellaril®; Stelazine®)

Haloperidol (Haldol®)

Lithium

Antidepressants (Elavil®; other tricyclic compounds)

- Other Frequently-Prescribed Drugs

Digitalis-digoxin (Lanoxin®)

Analgesics (codeine and related compounds)

Antihypertensives (especially beta blockers)

Drugs for diabetes

Cimetidine (Tagamet®)

Methyldopa (Aldomet®)

Propranolol (Inderal®)

Drugs having significant anticholinergic effects (belladonna; Probanthine®; pills or patches for seasickness)

Antihistamines (in many nonprescription formulas for allergy, colds and sleep)

Eye drops for glaucoma (especially beta blockers)

The subtle and unrecognized effects of medication on memory and other functions are illustrated by the severe fatigue, low blood pressure, and slowed pulse due to eye drops containing beta blockers. I have repeatedly encountered this problem, especially when another beta blocker was being prescribed concomitantly for hypertension or heart disease by a second physician.

MINIMIZE HABITS AND ACTIVITIES INVOLVING EXPOSURE TO OTHER POTENTIAL NEUROTOXINS AND SENSITIZING CHEMICALS
(Chapters 9, 11, 12 and 18)

- Avoid or limit alcohol consumption

Even small amounts should be avoided by persons who evidence consider able susceptibility to its effects (e.g., confusion and severe drowsiness)

Woman who are pregnant or attempting to become pregnant should not drink

The fetal alcohol syndrome, with lifelong severe learning defects and behavior disorders, more than tripled between 1979 and 1992

- Do not sniff inhalants

- Avoid or minimize pesticide residues in food (see above)

- Avoid exposure to pesticides and herbicides at home as much as possible

172

In the workplace
On golf courses
For lawn care
Growing food

- Avoid <u>other chemicals in the workplace</u> (industry; hospitals; offices; studios) <u>and in hobbies</u>

	E.g., exposure to solvents by painters, varnishers and carpetlayers, and industrial glues

- Avoid <u>smoking</u> (carbon monoxide; other noxious inhalants)

	The risk of AD may be increased up to fourfold among heavy smokers

- Avoid inhaling <u>perfumes, hairsprays, and other volatile fumes from toiletries</u>

- Avoid using <u>talcum powder and other fine dusts</u> that can be breathed into the body

- <u>Attempt to avoid or reduce exposure to chemicals and other toxins in the home</u> by these additional precautions:

	Use solid wood products instead of particle board (composed of left-over wood chips and bark, bonded with a formaldehyde-based glue)

	Choose hard wood or tiled floors

	Choose solid wood cabinetry

	Request paints and wood stains that are citrus oil based rather than petroleum based

	Use natural-fiber carpeting without formaldehyde-based stain protectors

	Use latex paint that is free of odor-causing volatile organic compounds (V.O.C.s)

	Insist on an adequate number of operable windows in order to vent the toxic gases released by building materials, carpets, upholstery and drapes

	Avoid scented candles because of the outgassing, even when not lit

	Place air returns near external doors that are frequently opened

	Reduce mold and mildew in warmer climates by limiting the opening of doors and windows (to avoid overtaxing air-conditioning systems)

	Leave ceiling fans running most of the time (to reduce the accumulation of moisture in humid homes)

	Correct the source of moisture when identified (e.g., a water heater; a leaky roof; poorly maintained air-conditioning system)

	Fireplaces can be a source of considerable chemical and mold inhalation in the absence of a good draft (logs are preferably stored outside)

	Dry-cleaned clothes should be aired away from living areas <u>before</u> being worn or placed in a closet or clothes cabinet (the perchloroethylene used can be highly toxic)

MINIMIZE EXPOSURE TO CARBON MONOXIDE
(Chapter 11)

- Minimize exposure from vehicular exhausts

    NEVER run a car engine in an unventilated garage with the door shut

    Have a reliable mechanic check the car's exhaust system to detect any leaks that could result in carbon monoxide accumulation

    Close the door between the garage and house whenever a vehicle is running (to prevent carbon monoxide from entering the house)

    Keep the car windows slightly open while driving in dense traffic

    An air conditioner may not prevent carbon monoxide accumulation

    Close the air intake (vents) when driving in heavy traffic or in a tunnel to minimize the interior collection of carbon monoxide fumes

- Attempt to minimize carbon monoxide exposure from other sources

    Check for defective water heaters, furnaces, and unsafe space heaters

    Virtually all gas stoves leak gas

    The pilot light should be turned off, especially if in the vicinity of a bedroom

    Exercise caution when using kitchen stoves as an ancillary heating system

    Take precautions when burning wood for heat

    The wood should be dry hardwood

    The chimney and stovepipe must be cleaned regularly

    Avoid the indoor burning of charcoal briquets (as when electrical power supply is disrupted without adequate ventilation for exhausting fumes to the outside)

    Insure adequate ventilation indoors when using any gasoline-powered equipment and other industrial machinery

    E.g., gasoline-powered washers operating inside buildings (as in the case of devices used by farmers to clean swine farrowing or birthing barns)

    Check for deficient ventilation in highly insulated homes and buildings

    Air conditioning units must be checked and cleaned regularly

    Avoid prolonged stays in enclosed ice rinks

    Carbon monoxide is released from ice cleaning machines and heaters

    Take precautions against the improper use or defective maintenance of gas-generated lamps, ovens and stoves in poorly-ventilated recreational vehicles

- Exercise caution with paint removers that contain methylene chloride

    Its absorbed vapors are converted in the liver to carbon monoxide

174

- Store containers away from living quarters
- Minimize prolonged travel in newer large aircraft with reduced air recirculation (Chapter 12)

AVOID INTENSE AND PROLONGED VISUAL POLLUTION; MODIFY ARTIFICIAL LIGHTING REDUCE RADIATION EXPOSURE
(Chapter 16)

General Considerations

*Proper light can be viewed as a form of "nutrition" necessary for optimum health

*Some students of radiation effects continue to warn about leaking from microwaves ovens, and challenge the nutritional value of microwaved-cooked food

- As far as possible, try to work and read in natural light

    At work

    In the home

- Minimize wearing tinted glasses and sunglasses

    New types of eyeglasses and contact lens allow the eyes to be exposed to ultraviolet light, whereas neutral gray sunglasses and tinted contact lenses block it

    Full-spectrum ultraviolet transmitting eyeglasses and contact lenses are available (Younger Optics in Los Angeles; Westley-Jessen Company in Chicago)

- Minimize "light shock" during the night

    Use a small blue Christmas-tree light in the bedroom or hallway

- Avoid intense light and glare, including:

    Traffic and bright midday sun during lunch-hour breaks

    Dazzling visual displays (strobe lights) at rock concerts or other events

- Watch television as far removed from the set as possible (at least six feet)

    Do not allow children to sit near the set

- Set limits on television viewing by young children

    Encourage them to engage in outdoor activity during daylight, particularly in the summer months

- Obtain a screen for video display terminals (VDTs)
- Change any defective lights or fixtures, especially fluorescent lighting

    Handle any broken fluorescent light rods carefully, and dispose of them properly

    A full-spectrum Chromalus incandescent bulb is available

- Prefer new types of fluorescent lights that closely duplicate natural sunlight

    Full-spectrum fluorescent tubes with added ultraviolet light are available

    The initial full-spectrum lighting devised by Ott has been protected by the addition of cathode ray shielding to lower radiation emission, and to improve the length of the ultraviolet component

    Consider investing in sunlight-simulating, full-spectrum lamps for schools and offices (*The Wall Street Journal* December 31, 1992, p. B-2)

- Remain alert to other forms of "radiation stress" including:

    Exposures to microwaves, radar systems, and radio or television antennas

    Avoid standing before microwave ovens when in use

    Medical radiation

    Close proximity to home entertainment centers and video arcades

    Electrical appliances on or immediately adjacent to the bed (blankets; clocks)

ENCOURAGE ACTIVITIES AND PRECAUTIONS THAT ENSURE ADEQUATE BRAIN OXYGENATION
(Chapter 12)

- <u>Attempt to breathe more deeply and regularly</u>

    Most adults breathe only at a fraction of their capacity, especially while concentrating

    A simple precaution for counteracting shallow breathing, especially among persons who do not exercise regularly, is taking several deep breaths on arising and intermittently during the day

    Such retraining can be done in conjunction with exercise (see below) and relaxation techniques (Chapter 19)

    The ensuing improved exchange of gases enables better oxygenation, more efficient release of gaseous waste products, and the greater receptivity and assimilation of information

- <u>Do not smoke</u>

- <u>Avoid prolonged sleep</u> (i.e., eight or more hours)—whether due to habit, narcolepsy, or sedatives and tranquilizers

- Consider <u>donating blood periodically</u> if polycythemia ("rich blood") exists

    It may reduce the tendency to both thrombosis and the accumulation of excessive iron, which is neurotoxic (Chapter 9)

    Many older persons with relatively high iron (ferritin) stores are good candidates as regular blood donors (Garry 1992)

- INSIST upon receiving oxygen in the immediate postoperative period to avoid the risk of hypoxemia (decreased blood oxygenation) (Chapter 12)

This precaution is especially important if coronary or cerebral vascular disease exists

• Avoid extreme and prolonged motions of the neck

Arching it backward, or twisting it sharply from side to side, can compress the vertebral arteries coursing through its vertebrae that carry one-fourth of the brain's blood supply

Examples of extreme positions:

Shampoos in beauty parlors and barber shops

Prolonged dental work

Prolonged painting of ceilings

Extreme chiropractic manipulations

Excessive arching by anesthesiologists prior to inserting a breathing tube

Such neck positions may be conducive to stroke in the presence of other medical risk factors (hypertension; diabetes), and local skeletal changes (arthritis; malformations)

• Follow recommendations for minimizing sleep apnea if present
This condition describes periodic prolonged nonbreathing, usually terminated by heavy snoring

• Comply with general prophylactic measures and medication for avoiding the vasospasm of migraine (Chapter 12)

• Minimize and compensate for prolonged air travel

Especially in newer large aircraft with reduced air recirculation (Tolchin 1993) (Chapter 12)

The adverse effects of "jet lag" induced by crossing three or more time zones can be reduced by adopting a sleep/wake schedule similar to the new location, and spending time outdoors the first few days (sunlight assists in synchronizing one's "internal clock")

• Special precautions by patients with chronic lung disease who risk hypobaric hypoxemia

Minimize air travel (Dillard 1991)

Gradually acclimatize to high-altitude facilities (e.g., ski lodges; alpine resorts)

CHALLENGE THE BRAIN TO ENHANCE ITS MEMORY BANKS, AND PRESERVE ADAPTIVE RESPONSIVENESS BOTH TO STRESS AND NEW INFORMATION
(Chapters 16 and 19)

General Considerations

*Such cognitive reinforcement during adult life favors continued branching of nerve cells, new nerve interconnections, and an increase of cholinergic neurons (Chapters 5 and 16)—the "use it or lose it" principle

*Awareness that physical and mental "death" may begin when one bemoans his or her "decline," and retreats by "giving up," might serve as a sobering antidote before and after retirement

*Many have found that the best secret to preserving youth is ongoing learning, exploring and experimenting.

> Harry Emerson Fosdick: "It is magnificent to grow old, if one keeps young."

• Emphasize mental activity through ongoing involvement in one's occupation, hobbies, travel, and educational pursuits ("mental calisthenics")… especially problem solving

There are numerous opportunities for continuing education

Adult classes given by local colleges and other teaching institutions (including museums)

Nature study groups

A large assortment of personal study programs offered by libraries

Elderhostel programs

Group travel can provide mental stimulation and exercise that counter the tendency to become more isolated as relatives and friends retire or become ill

Many organizations cater to special travel demands

• "Brain exercises" to "stretch the mind" may help retain or improve "working" memory

Practicing arithmetic without using a calculator

Various memory game-tests

Trying to write with either hand

Learning a foreign language

Playing a musical instrument

Painting

Doing woodwork

REMAIN PHYSICALLY ACTIVE DURING "MIDDLE AGE"

<u>General Considerations</u>

*There is increased awareness that exercise can reverse many changes associated with "aging"

*The benefits include increased muscle tissue, reduced fat, a lowered red blood cell count, reduced tendency to clot, decreased blood cholesterol and triglyceride concentrations, less loss of calcium from bone, and improved sugar-insulin metabolism

Exercise markedly improves functions essential for physical fitness in the elderly (Astrand 1992)

Exercise may minimize or prevent non-insulin-dependent diabetes mellitus (Manson 1992)

*The benefits of improved aerobic fitness include:
>   Quicker reaction times
>   Better recollection of names
>   Improved ability to solve arithmetic problems, and to perform other
>   mental tasks
>   Lessened tendency to depression

• <u>Engage in modest physical activity</u>—especially aerobic exercise and muscle strength training for 15-40 minutes, at least three times a week

>   Such aerobic exercise could consist of running, swimming, cycling, dancing, or walking briskly (3.5 miles per hour) after gradual training

• <u>Take proper precautions</u>

>   Exercise should be preceded by a "warm up" through gradual stretching, and followed by a gradual "cool down"

>   Avoid exhaustion, the lifting of excessive weights, or unduly painful stretching

>   Also take a brief midday <u>rest period or nap</u> as part of a preventive "wellness" program

>   >   The <u>siesta</u> long has been appreciated by Mediterranean, Latin and Asian societies

OPTIMIZE EMOTIONAL FUNCTIONS AND INTERPERSONAL RELATIONSHIPS
(Also see Chapter 19)

• <u>Partake of the activities and cognitive input of a high-functioning spouse</u>

• <u>Maintain sexuality</u> within reasonable and responsible bounds

• <u>Preserve close friendships</u>

• <u>Encourage continuing intergenerational relationships</u>

>   Avoid hostile or impulsive activities that tend to undermine them (Chapter 19)

• <u>Seek treatment for depression</u> (Chapters 13 and 16)

>   Especially if it has become a burden to personal health

PATIENTS AT HIGH RISK FOR STROKE AND VASCULAR DEMENTIA SHOULD HEED PRECAUTIONS AND TAKE PRESCRIBED MEDICATION

<u>General Considerations</u>

>   *Patients at high risk include smokers, the elderly, and persons with hypertension, diabetes, various forms of heart disease (especially atrial fibrillation), and transient ischemic attacks due to carotid (neck) arterial disease (Hachinski 1992)

- Stop smoking

- Exercise regularly

- Follow a diet to control diabetes, obesity, and excessively high blood cholesterol or triglycerides levels

- Minimize the use of salt

- Faithfully take antihypertensive drugs as directed

> But avoid severe declines of blood pressure

- Utilize non-pharmacologic measures as adjuncts to control hypertension

> Weight loss
>
> Rest periods
>
> Stress management (Chapter 19)

- Consult with your doctor about taking a "blood thinner," such as one aspirin every one or two days (if not medically contraindicated)

> Prescription anticoagulant drugs—coumarin (Coumadin®); dipyridamole (Persantine®)
>
> The anti-inflammatory effects of a small daily dose of aspirin may reduce reactions triggered by excitotoxins

- Consider carotid endarterectomy to remove obstructing plaques from the carotid (neck) arteries IF recommended by *several* knowledgeable physicians

UTILIZE PERTINENT GENETIC INFORMATION TO MINIMIZE NEUROTOXIC RISK

- Relatives of aspartame reactors and patients with Alzheimer's disease (Chapters 9 and 18)

> Avoid products containing aspartame (NutraSweet®)

- Phenylketonuria (PKU) carriers (Chapter 9)

> Minimize phenylalanine intake, especially as aspartame-containing products

- Galactosemia carriers (Chapters 9 and 18)

> Avoid excessive milk and milk products (including yogurt)
>
> Also avoid large amounts of certain fruits and vegetables that contain considerable galactose
>
>> E.g., apple; banana; Brussels sprouts; dates; papaya; tomato; watermelon

- Patients and families with lactose intolerance (Chapters 9 and 18)

> Minimize the amount of lactase added to milk, which may result in the excessive absorption of galactose

CAREFULLY WEIGH THE POTENTIAL BENEFIT AND HAZARDS OF NEW OR EXPERIMENTAL DRUGS THAT ALLEGEDLY PREVENT OR STABILIZE ALZHEIMER'S DISEASE

<u>General Considerations</u>

*Examples—chelating agents; excitotoxin blockers
- Chelation can remove neurotoxic metals—including lead, aluminum, mercury, cadmium and iron

*It will take <u>years</u> to evaluate the efficacy and safety of any "magic bullet" for humans with suspected proneness to AD
- Based on risk factors, changes by imaging studies (Chapter 4), or N-acetyl-L-aspartate (NAA) as a possible marker for neuronal degeneration (Klunk 1991, 1992)

18

PREVENTIVE NUTRITION

*Premature old age frequently occurs in people who live a
sedentary life, and at the same time consume much
rich food and alcohol.**

Dr. Arnold Lorand
(*Old Age Deferred* 1910, p. 107)

*There is growing interest in formulated foods that are termed
"prescriptive foods," "nutraceutical foods," or "designer foods"
... As much as these new developments may prove
beneficial, they also will provide opportunities for
confusion. Consumers will have to be ever
vigilant about the soundness
of health claims.***

Beatrice Trum Hunter (1991)

*There is no doubt in my mind that most of the common diseases
depend upon food for cause and cure save those from wounds,
injuries, contagion and infection... Patients, cooks and
almost all the laity are not willing to deny their appetites,
and had rather eat and die than eat to live.*

Dr. Ephraim Cutter (1893)

This chapter is devoted to prophylactic dietary practices and precautions. It is my conviction that proper food composition, preparation and intake are basic to any program whose goal is the prevention or delay of Alzheimer's disease (AD). While several aspects are raised apparently for the first time, this concept is not new.

- In *Noah's Planting*, Philo observed: "But the cooks and confectioners of our time… are always building up the senses with some new color, shape, scent or flavor, so as to utterly destroy the most important part of us, the mind."

- At the turn of this Century, Dr. Arnold Lorand (1910) (see introductory quote) recommended a diet "consisting of little meat, much milk, and vegetables" in a chapter titled, "The Rational Prevention of Premature Old Age and the Treatment of Old Age." He discouraged excessive use of tea and coffee, as well as a strictly vegetarian diet. Moreover, he did not regard wine as "the milk of old age."

Certain undesirable aspects of the contemporary diet were considered earlier. They include the aggravation of "functional" hyperinsulinism by high intake of sugar, concentrated carbohydrate and excessive protein (Chapter 8), and the neurotoxicity of certain additives (Chapter 9). The following aspects will be discussed here:

- The selection of desirable foods whenever it is possible to make such choices

- The safe preparation of foods

- Certain precautions during pregnancy and childhood

- The potential hazards of intentional semi-starvation, especially by young women who have an irrational morbid fear of obesity

GENERAL DIETARY PRECAUTIONS

I. Limit Sugar (Sucrose) and Refined Sugars (e.g., Fructose, Corn Syrup); Emphasize Complex Carbohydrates

The adverse effects of excessive simple sugars were reviewed in Chapters 7 and 8. Accordingly, complex carbohydrates (whole grains, vegetables, fruits, legumes) should account for a significant part of dietary calories… perhaps 50 percent or more for over-weight persons.

The "fine print" and slogans on labels—e.g., "diet"; "lite"; "low-calorie"; "sugar-free"; "cholesterol-free"—tend to be misleading. For example, "unsweetened" prune juice and grape juice still contain considerable "natural" sugar.

II. Consume Moderate Amounts of Protein and Amino Acids

The limited consumption of meat, chicken, lamb and fish—viz., three or four ounces per serving for an adult—is prudent. (Three ounces correspond in size to one quarter of an average-sized dinner plate, a deck of cards, or the palm of an average woman's hand.) Pork and products containing pork (e.g., hot dogs; sausages; deli meats) are best avoided. Vegetable sources of protein, such as whole grains and beans, should be used more abundantly.

Another dividend from such restraint relates to possible prevention of certain types of cancer, notably in the bowel. Whole grains and beans are known to increase the formation within the intestine of lignans and isoflavonoids, substances that may inhibit or slow the growth of tumor cells.

In contrast, <u>excessive</u> protein and amino acids (especially their uncommon D stereoisomers) can adversely affect brain function (Chapters 7 and 9) and accelerate the aging process. (Also see below)

- Impairment of liver and kidney functions is conducive to elevated concentrations of phenylalanine and other neurotoxic amino acids, both in the blood and brain.

- Although a high protein diet is prescribed routinely for persons prone to reactive hypoglycemia (Chapter 8), excessive amounts of protein could aggravate this condition by stimulating insulin release.

Excessive protein from meat and dairy products is also closely linked with excess fat intake. Accordingly, the use of more protein from vegetables, nuts, whole grains and beans is prudent.

III. <u>Avoid Excessive Calories</u>

Overeating, and the resulting gain in weight, enhance the risk of several metabolic and cardiovascular disorders that are conducive to AD, stroke and other health problems. They include severe hypoglycemia (Chapter 8), and elevated blood cholesterol and triglycerides (fat) levels. Hyperinsulinism is reduced by adhering to a prudent diet and avoiding excessive weight, especially among women (Wing 1992).

IV. <u>Avoid Foods Cooked at Very High Heat</u>

Cooking meat and other foods at high temperatures is undesirable (Chapter 7) due to the loss of many important enzymes. Overheated meat also generates heterocyclic amines that are suspected of causing cancer (Felton 1991).

Food processed by the following methods should be avoided or minimized (Hunter 1984):

- Frying, especially deep-fat frying
- Smoking—including fish (lox, salmon, whitefish, mackerel); poultry (turkey); bologna; cheese products (provolone); vegetables; fruits
- Dark roasting, charring and burning
- Using charcoal, wood and gas as fuels for grilled and barbecued foods
- Non-enzymic browning (the Maillard reaction)

The following practices are sensible:

- Select lean cuts of meat for grilling.
- Do not allow grilled food to become blackened and charred.
- Request beef that is "medium" rather than "well done"—but not "rare" or "medium rare."
- Use moist heat with steaming, simmering, stewing, boiling, poaching or microwave cooking—especially for foods of animal origin.

184

- Lower the heating temperature, but increase the cooking time.

- Avoid heating unsaturated oils, which promotes peroxidation. Olive oil, canola oil or butter are more stable.

PARAMETERS OF A "PROPER DIET"

The following foods are commonly available and less likely to cause or aggravate the undesired metabolic and neurotoxic effects noted earlier. The choices must be flexible owing to individual differences in both metabolism and food preferences.

I. Fruits

Most fresh and frozen unsweetened fruits are well tolerated. Excessively sweet fruits (e.g., mangos) and dried fruits (raisins; prunes; figs; dates) should be used sparingly, especially by persons subject to reactive hypoglycemia (Chapter 8).

Certain fruits and vegetables contain considerable galactose. They include apple, banana, Brussel sprouts, date, papaya, bell pepper, persimmon, pumpkin, tomato and watermelon (Gross 1991). If consumed in great quantity, they conceivably could be neurotoxic for individuals with the galactosemic trait (Chapter 9).

Sweetened commercial fruit juices and "fruit juice drinks" should be avoided. Raw juices (refrigerated) or 100% juices with no added sugar are preferable.

II. Vegetables

Most raw, fresh, frozen and home-canned vegetables prepared without additives are permissible. The ingestion of salads and vegetables, as well as whole grains and bran, also provides fiber.

By discarding the outer leaves of vegetables and peeling stone fruits (e.g., apples; pears; peaches), pesticide intake can be reduced.

Be vigilant to avoid sulfiting agents in restaurants. Although limited use is permitted for certain purposes, their presence must be declared on food labels.

III. Meats

Skinless chicken, turkey and lamb are the preferred choices. As noted above, they should be thoroughly cooked but not overheated ("well done").

Luncheon meats, sausage, ham and bacon should be avoided, or if used, eaten sparingly and infrequently.

IV. Milk and Dairy Products

Generally, milk, nonfat cottage cheese, plain yogurt, and soy products are tolerated by persons with a normal amount of lactase, an intestinal enzyme (Chapter 9). If obtainable, non-homogenized milk may have certain advantages over homogenized milk. All milk should be pasteurized for safety. (As many as 10 percent of dairy cattle in the United States are infected with *Campylobacter*.) Processed cheeses (American, Velveeta®) ought to be limited.

Cow's milk should not be given too early to infants. There may be immunologic reactions, with an increased risk of developing diabetes mellitus.

Butter, in moderate amounts, is probably preferable to margarine. The *trans* isomers of fatty acids, formed by the partial hydrogenation of vegetable oils to produce margarine and vegetable shortening, contribute to coronary heart disease—in part by increasing low-density-lipoprotein (LDL) cholesterol (Willett 1993).

V. Fish

Fish is a source of complete protein as well as desirable long-chain omega-3 fatty acids. Most fresh-water fish, salmon, water-packed tuna, and canned sardines from which the oil has been drained are acceptable. Fried fish and heavily salted fish are best avoided.

Certain large fish in tropical waters (e.g., kingfish, large grouper, red snapper and barracuda in South Florida; amberjack in Hawaii) should be avoided. They may contain the ciguatera neurotoxin, which is not destroyed by cooking or smoking.

> Ciguatera fish poisoning has become the most common seafood-related illness. There may be chronic neurologic symptoms (severe numbness and tingling; dizziness; blurred vision; protracted fatigue). The disorder results from ingesting the ciguatoxin present in fish that eat the reef feeders. (The toxin is produced by a protozoan organism which becomes attached to marine algae growing on coral reefs. It can cross the placenta and damage the fetus.) As a rule, yellowtail snapper and mahimahi are safe.

Because there are many species of fish, compared with domesticated animal foods, it is possible to eat a great variety. The benefit therein derives from limiting ingestion of the same toxins.

Unfortunately, concern about spoiled fish, and the contamination of fish by polychlorinated biphenyls (PCBs), mercury, other neurotoxic metals, and some pesticides has become necessary.

- Flounder and sole are generally free of pollutants.
- Salmon, white fish and swordfish often contain detectable amounts of PCBs.
- Clams occasionally are high in lead and cadmium.

VI. Grains

Most grains and grain products are satisfactory—provided much sugar has not been added, and they were not excessively processed (refined) such as white and "enriched" flour.

Whole wheat bread is best purchased from local health food stores that obtain it from small bakeries (especially when they avoid flour bleach).

Other whole grain products include rice, rye and buckwheat. Grains should be limited or avoided, however, if a clinical intolerance exists. This includes gluten intolerance, and the predictable occurrence of hypoglycemic attacks several hours after ingesting them… especially at breakfast.

White flour products tend to precipitate reactive hypoglycemia (Chapter 8). The presence of MSG and related substances (Chapter 9) also can cause problems.

Cornflakes and other cereals may contain considerable fluoride.

VII. Beans

If tolerated, most beans are satisfactory when cooked without added salt or animal fat.

VIII. Nuts

Most raw unsalted nuts, except peanuts, can serve as convenient snacks. Since nuts are concentrated foods, they should be eaten sparingly.

The peanut is not a true nut, but a legume. Even if well tolerated, peanuts should be consumed in moderation because they contain inhibitors of important enzymes.

Rancid or roasted nuts, and nuts exposed to air and light (as in showcases), should be avoided. Moldy peanuts may contain carcinogenic aflatoxins.

Roasting raw nuts and seeds in a warm oven tends to reduce the inhibitors of important enzymes.

IX. Soups

Many homemade soups (pea; vegetable; barley; onion; bean; lentil; brown rice) are wholesome, particularly when prepared without salt or fat.

Canned, creamed or dehydrated soups that contain manufactured monosodium glutamate (MSG) or hydrolyzed vegetable protein (HVP) (see below) should be avoided. The neurotoxic nature of these substances was discussed in Chapter 9.

X. Eggs

Gently simmered or poached eggs usually can be consumed in moderate amounts provided that there are no medical contraindications or other legitimate concerns. Some recommend "organic" eggs from range-free chickens not exposed to hormones, drugs or chemicals.

It is my belief that a slight elevation of the serum cholesterol concentration (according to current standards) does NOT justify total abstinence. The current promotion of costly "improved" eggs that allegedly do not elevate cholesterol levels should be viewed with skepticism. Moreover, they contain considerable vitamin E and iodine.

XI. Sweets and Sweeteners

Sugar, corn syrups, candy, and other conventional sugar products should be strictly limited—or better yet, avoided. Honey, maple syrup, and barley malt or rice syrup, if used as flavoring, should be used sparingly, especially by diabetics and persons subject to reactive hypoglycemia.

It is my opinion that the judicious use of *saccharin* is safe for most persons (Roberts 1989a, 1992b).

The neurotoxicity of *aspartame* was detailed in Chapter 9, and will be discussed below.

XII. Oils

Commercial oils are not natural foods. Virgin olive oil, unrefined oils, or even butter (see above) are preferable.

XIII. Snacks

Persons with diabetes and hypoglycemia (Chapter 8) require small feedings between meals and at night. Celery, carrots, radishes, low-carbohydrate fresh fruits, and unsalted and unroasted nuts and seeds can provide healthy and palatable snacks.

RESERVATIONS ABOUT ADDITIVES AND "SUPPLEMENTS"

The purported virtues and safety of many "natural" and "organic" products are constantly extolled for health-conscious persons. The potential hazards of several classes warrant reemphasis.

> Paracelsus, a famous physician in medical history, declared in his third "defension" (August 19, 1538): "Everything is a poison, the dose alone makes a thing not a poison."

This issue is rendered more complex by food idiosyncrasies and the so-called multiple chemical sensitivity (MCS) syndrome (Chapter 11). Severe brain reactions have been ascribed to trace amounts of chemicals used in common foods as colorings, flavorings and preservatives, and for other purposes.

I. Aspartame (NutraSweet®)

In my opinion, *most persons concerned about the risk of AD should deliberately avoid products containing aspartame.* This precaution extends to young children, pregnant women (see below), patients with anemia, liver disease or kidney disease, and PKU carriers.

The avoidance of such products is even more relevant for persons with impaired memory. The confusion and memory loss experienced by consumption of products containing aspartame were described in Chapter 9.

Persons who react adversely to aspartame products ALWAYS must remain alert to the unannounced substitution of aspartame for other sweeteners. This action by producers has occurred repeatedly—for example, the corporate decision to use up a supply of old labels on soft drinks after their reformulation with aspartame... but with no declaration of its presence on the label (Roberts 1989).

II. Monosodium Glutamate (Manufactured Glutamic Acid; MSG)

The neurotoxicity of MSG and related substances was reviewed in Chapter 9. This ubiquitous flavor intensifier is commonly "hidden" in foods products, candy, chewing gum, soft drinks, and binders for medication. Some of flavorings and seasonings that contain it are Accent®, Zest®, Subu®, Glutavene®, and Lawry's Seasoning Salt®.

The following guide for consumers of food label descriptors that are always or often associated with the presence of MSG in food products is modified after Dr. Adrienne Samuels (1991) (reproduced with permission):

- These ALWAYS contain MSG:

    Monosodium glutamate   Autolyzed yeast
    Hydrolyzed vegetable protein   Textured protein
    Sodium caseinate   Calcium caseinate
    Yeast extract
    Yeast nutrient

- These often contain MSG:

    Malt extract   Flavoring(s)
    Malt flavoring   Natural flavoring(s)
    Bouillon   Natural beef flavoring
    Barley malt   Natural chicken flavoring
    Broth   Natural pork flavoring
    Stock   Seasonings
    Tomato Paste

- These CREATE MSG:

    Protease enzymes   Protease
    Fungal protease

- These MUST BE REGARDED WITH SUSPICION

    Whey protein   Torula yeast
    Carrageenan   Smoke flavoring
    Soy protein isolate   Soy protein concentrate
    Whey protein concentrate Vegetable gum
    Enzymes   Yeast food
    Stock   Hydrolyzed oat flour

Individuals suspected of being sensitive to MSG must <u>constantly</u> check ALL labels, and question restaurant managers, to prevent recurrent "diagnosis by illness." Terms such as "no MSG added" and "all natural" do NOT exclude its presence. Moreover, reactions to MSG may not be dose related in the case of individuals who react to minute amounts. (Sensitivity is generally not a problem with glutamic acid or glutamate present in unadulterated protein.)

Hidden MSG is not limited to foods. MSG-sensitive persons have reported reactions caused by soaps, shampoos, hair conditioners, and cosmetics that contain MSG, especially as "hydrolyzed protein" or "amino acids." Binders of medications, nutrients and supplements—both prescription and non-prescription—also may contain MSG.

III. <u>Synthetic Food Colorings and Flavorings</u>

Synthetic food colorings and flavorings have a poor history of safety. A number that were thought to be safe at one time had to be banned later. Even many of those in use at present are of doubtful safety.

Whenever possible, concerned consumers should avoid synthetically colored and flavored foods and beverages. They include sodas, smoked salmon, margarine and diet spreads.

The same caution applies to other synthetically colored and flavored products—viz., drugs, vitamins, and toiletries such as tooth pastes, mouth washes and cough syrup.

IV. Amino Acids

The potential adverse effects on neurotransmitter function (Chapter 5) of many individual amino acids that are commercially available were noted in Chapter 7. Extensive marketing of these products continues. Some are touted as potential cures for medical disorders. Other promotionals allege that they "increase the arousal index," or "inhibit an enzyme that breaks down brain endorphins and enkephalins."

Virtually all the essential amino acids have been recommended for treating stress and poor memory. Such capricious use by consumers, however, should be discouraged… particularly AD-prone individuals.

As a case in point, amino acids—alone or in combination "amino acid cocktails"—are being recommended to enhance or "jump-start" brain function. These "smart drugs" include phenylalanine, tryptophan, arginine, ornithine, and related products (e.g., melatonin; vasopressin; pyroglutamate).

> One popular "nutritional beverage mix" for increasing energy contains 600 mg L-phenylalanine per tablespoon. The label suggests up to four tablespoons daily; this would total 2,400 mg L-phenylalanine!

Phenylalanine and other amino acids stimulate insulin release (Floyd 1966, 1970; Reitano 1978). Accordingly, they may be detrimental for persons subject to hypoglycemia (Chapter 8).

The hazard of ingesting single amino acids, with or without neurotoxic contaminants, has been dramatically illustrated by the eosinophilia-myalgia syndrome following use of L-tryptophan. This serious disorder, mainly experienced by women, is characterized by severe muscle and joint pains, fatigue, a rash, swelling, involvement of multiple nerves (polyneuropathy), and a striking elevation of the blood eosinophil count.

V. Vitamins and Minerals

One or two standard multivitamin pills or capsules may be beneficial for active adults, especially when the timing and nature of their meals are unpredictable. Deficiencies (an intake of less than two-thirds the Recommended Daily Allowances) are often encountered in the general population, especially among the elderly.

- The more frequent deficits include folic acid, vitamin B-6 (pyridoxine), vitamin B-12, vitamin D, calcium, magnesium, chromium and zinc—but generally not vitamin E.

- Some deficiencies induce a decline in cognitive function, which can be prevented or reversed with modest doses (Rosenberg 1992).

- Joosten et al (1993) provided further evidence that deficiencies of vitamin B-12, folic acid and pyridoxine commonly occur in elderly persons. Lindenbaum et al (1994) emphasized that many elderly persons are "metabolically deficient in cobalamin or folate" even though their serum vitamin concentrations are "normal." Intracellular deficiency of these vitamins is evidenced by the elevation of important metabolites (homocysteine, cystathionine, methylmalonic acid,

2-methylcitric acid) that are dependent on adequate concentrations of these vitamins.

- Elevation of homocysteine appears to favor premature occlusive vascular disease (Selhub 1993).

The **B vitamins** are present in dairy products, meats, dried beans and peas, and other foods. Vitamin B-6 is plentiful in bananas and avocados. There is considerable vitamin B-12 in beef and clams.

The <u>supplementary use</u> of the following individual vitamins in prudent daily doses is reasonable.

- **Vitamin B-1** (thiamine) (50-100mg) by individuals who habitually drink alcohol.

- **Vitamin B-6** (pyridoxine) (100 mg), but preferably as pyridoxal-5-phosphate (50mg)—especially in the "detoxification" of persons found to have elevated aluminum levels in hair or urine. Pyridoxine deficiency can enhance the toxicity of MSG (*Nutrition Reviews* 1973; 31(2): 70-71).

- **Vitamin B-12** for vegetarians who do not consume meat or fish.

- **Vitamin C** (ascorbic acid). There is considerable evidence, including double-blind studies, that vitamin C is helpful in both the treatment and prevention of various diseases. An optimal amount generally can be achieved by taking 500 mg vitamin C once or twice daily—approximately equivalent to 12 glasses of orange juice. (In view of the water-soluble nature of vitamin C and its prompt elimination by the kidneys, some have suggested that it be ingested several times daily.)

   An estimated 400 mg vitamin C—about seven times the Recommended Daily Allowance (RDA)—is required daily for maintaining general health. Yet, only nine percent of adults attain adequate levels through the consumption of five servings of fruit and vegetables daily to satisfy the current recommended requirement of 60 mg vitamin C. There is need for considerably more vitamin C by persons who smoke and who drink alcohol. Moreover, marginal or severe hypovitaminosis C (determined by its concentration in the buffy coat layer of blood) is the rule among institutionalized patients.

   Some physicians are impressed by the improvement of fatigue and cerebration with supplemental vitamin C, based on clinical observation and concomitant studies of cognitive function. There also are numerous references to improved periodontal disease and dental caries, greater resistance to infection, increased capillary strength, and better diabetic control with supplemental vitamin C.

   Dosages of 2,000 mg or more have been recommended for the "detoxification" of persons with elevated aluminum levels in hair or urine.

Chromium may benefit persons with hypoglycemia and diabetes through its effect on insulin metabolism. There is considerable chromium in whole grains, liver, poultry, beef, unprocessed fruits, vegetables, potatoes (with skin), and brewer's yeast. Supplemental chromium picolinate (200 micrograms daily) could be taken for the aforementioned conditions, and as a safe "anti-aging" substance (Passwater 1993).

- Trivalent chromium helps insulin move nutrients through the cell membrane and into cells for maintenance, repair and replication. It also appears to protect against glycation, a process involving the reaction of glucose and fructose with collagen and other proteins that results in the stiffening of tissues.

- The picolinic acid aids in the absorption of chromium and zinc from food.

Supplementary **zinc** may restore or boost the aging immune system (Good 1993). An intake of 50-60 mg oral zinc gluconate or zinc sulfate per day is the equivalent of 15 mg elemental zinc. Most of the enzymes involved in replication of immune cells require zinc, as does synthesis of thymic humoral factor. But high concentrations might precipitate brain amyloid (*Science* 1994; 265:1464-1467).

Magnesium protects nerve cells from the energy depletion and vulnerability to free radicals and excitotoxins associated with its deficiency due to poor diet, alcohol, disease and drugs. It is abundant in green leafy vegetables, whole grains, nuts, meat, poultry and fish. Various magnesium salts are available as supplements. They include magnesium taurate, magnesium potassium taurate, magnesium oxide-adenosine triphosphate, and solutions of magnesium chloride and acetate.

Smith (1993) reported that the concentrations of most elements in "**organically**" **grown fruits and vegetables**—on a fresh weight basis—averaged about twice (!) that of commercial foods of similar variety and size. These analyses by state-of-the-art instruments suggest several possibilities, including the importance of post-harvest handling.

Chapter 17 listed **caveats concerning the use and abuse of vitamins and minerals**. Much of the hype and inferences about the value of <u>megadose</u> vitamin-mineral therapy is not only misleading but also potentially harmful. Dr. Lita Lee (1990) wrote in her *Radiation Protection Manual*:

> "It is not wise to take megadoses of isolated nutrients, such as a single B vitamin, a single amino acid, high doses of ascorbic acid without the rest of the complex, high doses of vitamin E, etc. Why? You should know that the nutrient that controls your body chemistry is the one in lowest amount, not the one you are megadosing."*

The possible <u>adverse effects of excessive vitamin E and iron overload</u> warrant special attention.

- **Vitamin E.** There is widespread over-medication with this fat-soluble vitamin, which is abundant in vegetable oils, wheat germ oils, whole grains, sunflower seeds, almonds and other foods. The RDA is 10-15 international units (IU). At least one-fourth of adults in the United States now consume megadoses—400 IU or more daily—for its alleged therapeutic or preventive effects, largely resulting from enormous promotion and marketing. Hypovitaminosis E is rare, however, occurring chiefly in premature babies and persons with severe malabsorption problems.

  In my opinion, the ability of vitamin E to function as an "antioxidant" in destroying "free radicals" has been projected to extremes by nutritionists, the wellness press, medical periodicals and corporate interests. (Vitamin E also may function as a pro-oxidant). There is even the inference that megadoses can prevent or retard senility ("Project Methuselah").

Unfortunately, hypervitaminosis E can be serious. I have reviewed its complications (Roberts 1979b, 1981c, 1984b, 1993c). They include hypertension, thrombophlebitis, pulmonary embolism, breast tumors, altered immunity, and severe fatigue.

- **Iron.** Iron can be neurotoxic (Chapter 11). It accumulates within vital areas of the brain in both AD and Parkinson's disease. The FDA is considering a reduction in the recommended daily allowance of iron from 18 mg to 12 mg. (As reference, one bowl of Kellogg's Product 19® contains 18 mg iron.)

VI. Choline and Lecithin

Other related substances that might be beneficial, and are unlikely to have serious side effects, could be used by concerned persons with multiple AD risk factors. They include choline (a component of acetylcholine), which is present in concentrated lecithin.

DIETARY PRECAUTIONS DURING AND AFTER PREGNANCY

Adhering to a proper diet during and after pregnancy as prophylaxis against AD for the offspring might seem a strange idea. Yet, that is when the preventive effects of proper nutrition begin to influence brain function—and the subsequent quality of life—most profoundly. For example, severe restriction of calories, protein, or both, during pregnancy is known to decrease the number of brain cells present at birth (Winick 1970).

A listing of the more important dietary suggestions appears at the beginning of Chapter 17. The unique value of breast milk for proper brain development merits further discussion.

Avoidance Of Aspartame

I have stressed the potential problems from consuming food and beverage products that contain aspartame during pregnancy (Roberts 1989a, 1992b), particularly the adverse effects of phenylalanine and methyl alcohol.

- Pregnancy limits the conversion of phenylalanine to tyrosine (Yakymyshyn 1972).

- Increased concentrations of phenylalanine during the third trimester could interfere with brain and body development.

- Cleft lip and cleft palate occur more frequently with elevated phenylalanine levels (Tocci 1973).

The Importance of Breast-Feeding

The desirability of breast-feeding, and the shortcomings of arbitrary bottle-feeding, cannot be overemphasized. A mother's milk has vast advantages over commercial infant formulas—notably optimum brain and nerve development, and providing significant immunity against infection. Unfortunately, the promotion and use of infant formulas have severely undermined the practice of breast-feeding in "developed" countries.

In addition to the long-chain lipids critical for structural development of the nervous system, human milk has numerous hormones and trophic factors that influence brain growth and maturation. On the other hand, there is potential damage by "unnatural" formula feeding in early infancy relative to abnormal neural development and function.

- Breast-milk cholesterol is important for optimizing development of the myelin sheath that envelops nerve cells (Anderson 1973).

- Pre-term infants fed mother's milk (even by tube) gain significant benefit in terms of neural development and their subsequent intelligent quotient (IQ). This phenomenon is still detectable eight years later (Lucas 1992).

NUTRITION IN INFANCY AND CHILDHOOD

Insuring the proper nutrition of children is essential in the prevention of neurological and developmental disorders. Conversely, malnutrition can adversely affect cellular proliferation during the first six months (Winick 1970).

A listing of important dietary precautions for children appears in Chapter 17. Excessive calories, sugar and additives (e.g., high-sugar "reconstituted" drinks; sugary breakfast cereals) are especially damaging for young children prone to severe hypoglycemia and hyperactivity (Chapter 8).

The Issue of Intentional Malnutrition

I regard with dismay the intentional underfeeding of young children by "sophisticated" parents who hope to prevent coronary heart disease, dental caries, cancer, and other degenerative disorders thereby.

This misguided idea derives from studies demonstrating increased longevity in animals whose caloric, carbohydrate and protein intake had been reduced during the neonatal period. Unfortunately, children cannot completely "catch up" with the lessened number of brain cells induced by malnutrition during the fetal stage or infancy.

THE "FEAR OF FAT" ISSUE

Arbitrary and excessive restriction of calories should be avoided by children and young adults because of its potential long-term complications, especially on brain development and function, as well as psychological damage. Sadly, "fear of fat" permeates our society (Roberts 1989a, 1992b). This obsession frequently plagues both boys and girls. It is most pernicious among young women of essentially normal weight who attempt to simulate the bodies of starved actresses and models.

In a survey of 364 female college freshmen, Frank et al (1991) found that 60 percent were on a diet to lose or maintain lower weight. Moreover, at least 29 percent used crash dieting or fasting to achieve this goal since entering college seven months earlier. Twenty percent resorted to diet pills, and 13 percent had used some method of purgative—including vomiting, laxatives, and diuretics.

This issue is underscored by the apparent increased vulnerability of women to AD (Chapter 16). Their loathing of "those five extra pounds on my thighs" (Roberts 1992b) constitutes a significant risk factor. These same fatty deposits actually constitute important energy reserves, reflecting the "thrifty gene" that enabled ancestors to survive during periods of starvation (Chapter 8).

I have reviewed the medical and neurologic tragedies resulting from irrational caloric restriction (Roberts 1970b, 1985). They include the precipitation of severe headache (Roberts 1967a), heart disorders (Roberts 1967a), thyroid problems (Roberts 1969a), emotional disturbances, gallstones, and attacks of multiple sclerosis (Roberts 1966b,c).

Since brain changes initiated in this manner could antedate AD, they should be cause for concern and proper advice by parents, teachers and physicians.

19

*PREVENTIVE TECHNIQUES TO COPE WITH STRESS**

The whole secret of remaining young in spite of years, and even of gray hairs, is to cherish enthusiasm in one's self by poetry, by contemplation, by charity—that is, in fewer words, by the maintenance of harmony in the soul.

Henri Frederic Amiel
(*Journal Intime* 1874)

All knowledge is in the human mind, but it remains covered. Learning is the process of uncovering the veil that shrouds knowledge...We have to know how to act. We must remember that the intent of all work is simply to bring out the power of the mind which is already there to be awakened.

Swami Vivekananda

---

*A three-cassette set on this subject, discussed by H.J. Roberts, M.D., is available from The Sunshine Sentinel Press, Inc. P.O. Box 8697, West Palm Beach, FL 33407; FAX (407) 832-2400, $24.95. It is titled, *A Guide to Personal Peace: The Control of Stress, Anxiety, Worry and Depression.*

This chapter addresses another long-term strategy to prevent or minimize Alzheimer's disease (AD): constructive attitudes and coping mechanisms likely to reduce the effects of stress and emotional overload that contribute to AD (Chapter 13). They supplement the "physical" and "medical" recommendations listed in Chapters 17 and 18. Stress reduction, coupled with other attributes of both conventional and alternative medicine that enable persons to live in harmony with whatever level of health or illness they have been experiencing, is known to facilitate "healing of the mind" (Moyers 1993).

Severe anxiety, chronic tension, and feelings of inability to cope with stress influence neuromediators (Chapter 5), and even can impair immune responses (Chapter 6). Stein, Schiavi and Camerino (1976) stated: "Although clinicians now have an increased understanding of the immunological basis of a variety of illnesses, little attention has been paid to the psychophysiological aspects of the immune process." A pleasant event (e.g., family celebration; pursuing leisure activities; meeting with friends) has been shown to boost the immune system as long as two days (Stone 1994). Conversely, stressful encounters (especially at the work place) tend to have adverse effects— including susceptibility to colds.

Young adults evidence maturity whenever they seek the advice and guidance of respected individuals—be it a relative, friend, teacher, religious leader, physician, psychologist or social worker—on how to handle challenges encountered along life's unchartered road. Concomitantly, there is much gratification for those willing to assist them. Few personal gifts ensure lifelong gratitude more than that accorded persons who offer such insights learned from their own experiences. Hopefully, this section will help in the effort.

Reference was made in Chapters 17 and 18 to the brain's inherent recuperative powers when damaging dietary and other neurotoxic influences are avoided or controlled. These powers also can be mobilized during "the harvest years" through continual mental stimulation, education, travel, other challenging activities, and healing philosophies. Although often demanding, the effort and discipline should be encouraged to avert the pathos of dementia.

The following attitudes and coping techniques have been culled from "the wisdom of the ages." They deserve serious consideration in an holistic approach to AD prevention. While there is no guarantee that they will prevent AD, these helpful adjuncts certainly can provide the means to achieving a fuller, enriched life.

LEARN TO CULTIVATE INNER PEACE FOR COPING WITH LIFE'S STRESSES

Tension and frustration are inevitable experiences, especially at strategic "passages" in life. Often these emotions are generated by problems associated with illness, child rearing, financial misfortune, strained family relationships, and concomitants of the aging process.

Wise persons have offered useful advice to anticipate and prepare for personal and societal turmoil in this "Age of Anxiety." President Herbert Hoover emphasized the value of creating "peace at the center" in order to cope. But "peace of mind" should not be equated with escape from responsibility, nor with denial of real hurts and injustices.

Fashion a personalized program for stress control.

There are relatively simple techniques that can contribute to mental serenity when one is confronted with heavy pressures. An effective program to control stress could include these components:

- Have faith in yourself, and trust in your own ability to cope with and adapt to crises. In a real sense, this power represents mankind's greatest heritage.

- When upset over "What-if… ?" situations, repeat these "five magic words": "I'll handle it when necessary!"

- Define the basic problem, and then be prepared to make any necessary changes—e.g., following recommended treatment for an illness, or adapting your life style to new conditions.

- Find ways to use your energies productively instead of brooding constantly on a problem, especially if it is largely imaginary.

- Do what you feel is right for you. Do not accept blindly what others think you ought to do.

- Make decisions only after thinking things through and seeking advice. If you feel pressured, use the lawyers' standard reply: "I'm taking it under advisement."

Take time for "purposeful pausing," even if only for brief relaxed contemplation, in order to break the vicious cycle of tension.

Daily periods of solitude afford the opportunity to reduce tension and encourage creative thinking. This has been termed "creative relaxation" (Blanton 1965).

During these islands of privacy, the brain can summon its remarkable abilities to lessen anxiety, coordinate thoughts in proper decision-making, and for healing. Henry Wadsworth Longfellow described the "success mechanism" of enlightened relaxation in *The Builders*.

> "Nothing useless is, or low;
> Each thing in its place is best;
> And what seems but idle show
> Strengthens and supports the rest."

Use the relaxation response.

Ultimately, each individual needs to find the best way to induce relaxation for preventing the buildup of tension and stress. Many have found the following techniques helpful.

- Seek a quiet environment without distractions or noise. An eye shade or ear plugs may be helpful.

- Assume a restful position in a comfortable chair or on a couch at some convenient time (often during a lunch break), and loosen any tight-fitting clothing. The head and the arms should be supported, the shoes removed, and the feet propped up several inches.

- Initiate the relaxation response by closing the eyes, and sequentially relaxing all muscles —beginning with the scalp and eyes, and progressing down the face, neck, upper extremities, torso and lower limbs. Or, work in the reverse order. At the outset, it is helpful to tighten particular groups of muscles in order to sense the ensuing relaxation more completely when they are unclenched.

198

- Initiate a steady breathing rhythm, preferably through the nose. As you breathe out, say "one" silently as a simple, neutral stimulus. Follow this by breathing in, and then breathing out, silently saying the word "two." Repeat each sequence to "four," and then resume with "one."

- Continue the exercise 15 to 20 minutes (preferably avoiding any external signaling from an alarm clock). Practice this procedure twice daily, if possible.

"Recharge your batteries."

Increase your energy and enthusiasm in a host of individualized ways. They include regular rest periods (see above), non-fatiguing exercise, listening to uplifting beautiful music, reading (generally re-reading) great works of literature, and enjoying the company of children, grandchildren, or the children of friends and neighbors.

Obtain adequate sleep, preferably without a sedative.

A state of physical exhaustion is not conducive to coping effectively with problems. Numerous studies indicate the hazards of sleep deprivation and the habitual use of sedatives—e.g., severe insomnia when they are stopped; sleep apnea with prolonged nonbreathing (Chapter 12). Often, techniques for stress reduction and relaxation (see above) induce better sleep.

Use "word therapy" as another effective technique.

Word therapy describes the conscious replacement of negative and destructive thoughts by certain words, phrases, favorite songs, religious hymns, lines of poetry, or word-pictures that predictably induce tranquility and comfort in an individual.

Think "positively," and banish constant thoughts of criticism.

What we think, we become. Accordingly, it is wise to avoid destructive negative thoughts and constant worry. An adage avers: "Thinking can get you out of a problem. Worry can get you into one." Also, remember what Mark Twain said: "All my life I've worried—about the wrong things!"

Another helpful perspective involves the truism that those who constantly criticize others probably are unhappy, disturbed, or both. The same applies to the warped utterances of ever-present "doom-mongers." Disraeli astutely observed that it is easier to be critical than correct.

Anticipate criticism, and be prepared to handle it sensibly.

This approach has enabled many creative individuals to endure ridicule and rejection. Otherwise, harsh criticism from a spouse, an in-law, a customer, or a boss could be devastating. On this subject, Abraham Lincoln noted:

> "If I tried to read, much less to answer, all the criticisms made of me and all the attacks leveled against me, this office would have to be closed for all other business. I do the best I know, the very best I can. I mean to keep on doing this, down to the very end."

One learns, from experience, that excessive or unwarranted criticism often gives a glimmer of the aforementioned suppressed unhappiness, rejection, or some other emotional disturbance within the critic who desperately attempts to ventilate it. Under these circumstances, such behavior ought not be interpreted as a personal affront. Also, it is helpful to recognize that love and hate can overlap in a person's feelings toward the same individual.

Learn to compromise.

Maturity teaches the imperative of proper compromise to attain "peace of mind." This means the acceptance of limitations—in family as well as in business and professional relationships.

Do not remain hostage to faulty memories.

Many persons have held themselves hostage to fantasies and illusions based on faulty memory. The ensuing regrets left in their wake about "what might have been"—be it a previous romance or lost opportunity—undermined their creative living forever after. Listen to T. S. Eliot in _Bornt Noron_.

> "Footfalls echo in the memory
> Down the passage which we did not take
> Towards the door we never opened
> Into the rose garden."

Learn the wisdom of forgiveness.

Carrying a grudge indefinitely, both against others and one's self, can undermine personal peace due to the enervating anxiety, fatigue and depression. They probably represent an alteration of neuromediators (Chapter 5).

The need for self-forgiveness is imperative. Persons who carry excessive and prolonged guilt over "what might have been" or "the good old days" show the aging effects of this burden in their facial expression, posture, and behavior.

The "wisdom of the ages" emphasizes the benefits of forgiveness, and of becoming "a judge without a grudge." Forgiveness, after all, is a thought by which one simply "lets go."

- Shakespeare recognized the value of both forgiveness and mercy in these lines from _The Merchant of Venice:_

  > "The quality of mercy is not strained;
  > It droppeth as the gentle rain from heaven
  > Upon the place beneath: it is twice blest—
  > It blesseth him that gives and him that takes."

- J. K. Lagemann (1965), a victim of Nazi brutality, expressed the benefit of forgiveness: "Unless you forgive, you cannot love. And without love, life has no meaning."

Avoid unwarranted self-criticism when you feel you did your best or simply made a wrong decision.

Unwarranted self-criticism is a form of self-flagellation I have repeatedly encountered among patients and friends. They criticize themselves mercilessly for some "mistake" of a personal, economic, professional or business nature. Continued disapproval, especially when accompanied by an inferiority complex and fear of the future, is likely to ensure the self-fulfilling prophecy of failure.

Verbalizing some perceived problem, along with a reasonable solution to "make a lemon into a lemonade," often results in the dissipation of conflict, or acceptance of the situation, without leaving a residual stigma or depression.

200

Accept realistically any shortcomings of your job or career.

Many persons consider changing their goals and occupations at "mid-life." I personally have known physicians who decided to make major changes, and then became full-time writers, businessmen, lawyers, artists, priests, and real estate developers.

Before making any drastic change, however, analyze all the reasons for being unhappy about your work or career. This kind of realistic exercise is imperative to avoid pursuing ill-conceived, unrealistic fantasies that promise "fulfillment." Seek professional help from individuals whose wisdom and objectivity you respect, and carefully study the advice before making any final decision.

Learn to verbalize righteous indignation.

The suppression of anger ("peace at any price") not only fails to eliminate the problem, but prevents both parties from confronting the real issues. Relationships have been often salvaged by expressing justified anger, and telling the offender why a hurt was experienced so deeply. Paradoxically, venting anger may make the offender realize that the indignant critic _really_ cares.

Dr. Rolland S. Parker (1973) suggested these guidelines to express anger properly:

- Try to understand all the issues involved.
- Confirm that the other person is indeed the one who provoked the emotion.
- Respond only when it is timely, and in a degree appropriate to the provocation.

Asserting one's legitimate rights—whether concerning defective goods, poor service, or abuse—is not being "overly aggressive." In fact, reacting in an assertive manner may generate high psychological dividends of increased self-esteem.

Respect your own creative ideas and skills.

The imaginative mind is a wellspring of original thought, whatever the subject… business, technology, or the arts. Individual insights beyond the routine and the conventional should be pursued despite anticipated criticism or denigration by others. Even with initial shortcomings, original ideas ultimately may lead to successful offshoots.

Expressing one's innate creativity is important for stimulating brain function. The chief ingredients are proper motivation, acquiring the necessary skills through education and practice, and regarding the enterprise as a noble path to personal fulfillment.

Develop the habit of writing down any ephemeral ideas promptly after they come. This may require keeping a note pad by the night stand. The subconscious mind often generates novel answers that are appropriate to some great challenge or conflict. They frequently surface during tranquil periods or the light sleep of "creative relaxation" (see above).

Recognize the pitfalls when fame and appreciation are sought.

Ambitious persons may be pulled into the quicksand of seeking fame. Although there is merit in the saying, "Nobody will blow your horn unless you do," the overaggressive pursuit of fame generally proves unproductive.

On the other hand, fame tends to reward creative work done with modesty, especially when the fruits of such labor are then donated to others—even at the risk of encouraging plagiarism. Of fame, Alexander Pope aptly wrote

> "Nor Fame I slight, nor for her favours call;
> Comes unlook'd for, if she comes at all."

Tap the fountain of your spiritual experience for leads and guidance to achieve "peace at the center."

Faith and prayer can be uniquely meaningful in a complex world when one experiences severe tension, stress and uncertainty. This truism has been enshrined for persons of all faiths in *Psalm 23:*

> "The Lord is my shepherd;
> I shall not want.
> He maketh me to lie down in green pastures;
> He leadeth me beside the still waters.
> He restoreth my soul."

Spiritual and philosophic teachings also serve to temper human drives and desires, especially in curbing the pursuit of ambition toward dangerous extremes. In our competitive and materialistic society, young adults are challenged to exercise their talents without becoming dehumanized or demoralized.

Valid spiritual experiences may influence brain physiology constructively. All religions aim to "awaken" within believers an awareness of the calling to be more perceptive to their own basic needs as well as those of society. Such is the purpose of techniques as brief voluntary fasts, blowing the Shofar, leading a service, and hearing inspired renditions by choirs.

Unfortunately, many persons must come to grips with certain religious dogmas that act as stumbling blocks to personal peace. The doctrine of "original sin," for example, might seem the antithesis of a loving and redeeming God.

ADOPT TENSION-REDUCING TECHNIQUES
TO HANDLE DAILY ACTIVITIES

Divide your day into small segments of effective time.

One cannot simultaneously address all the details of running a business or a profession or a home—e.g., returning phone calls; answering mail; doing numerous chores. Reduce tension by learning to handle and complete each task.

Make a list of your activities and tasks for the day, and establish priorities that differentiate between "urgent" and "important" tasks.

Most successful persons use this "to-do list" technique. Without it, various activities intrude… followed by the tension and confusion on recalling forgotten or uncompleted tasks. Fatigue and other adverse effects are likely to ensue.

Incorporate your natural habits and behavioral patterns into the daily schedule.

Striking individual differences exist in patterns of energy, sleep and other physiologic functions. There are "larks" and "owls." Some persons function most efficiently in the morning, while others achieve their maximum productivity during the afternoon or late evening.

Similarly, some can work on prolonged tasks seemingly without fatigue, while others require rest periods of varying duration to "recharge." These may include coffee or snack breaks, a visit to the restroom, or a brief nap.

Incorporate "safety valve" relaxation periods into your routine.

I previously advised setting aside blocks of the day, or perhaps a specific day, in order to catch up, relax in a "do-nothing chair," or engage in some form of recreation. This is especially helpful for work addicts ("workaholics").

"Safety valves" help to cope with pressure, and to lessen boredom and fatigue. They also encourage creative thoughts. Successful authors generally adopt variations of the "50-10" method—i.e., writing 50 minutes, and then resting or switching to another activity for 10 minutes.

Try the Benefits of Meditation.

There is widespread acceptance of the possible value to be derived from meditation in confronting daily stresses. This entails sitting quietly in a peaceful environment for 15-20 minutes in an effort to guide the mind to tranquility. It is not necessary to have a religious focus because concentration on some word, thought or feeling to prevent the mind from wandering can suffice. The mind tends to be more fresh and alert thereafter.

UTILIZE BASIC COMMUNICATION RULES FOR BETTER UNDERSTANDING AND PROMOTING FRIENDSHIPS

*Learn to recognize the feelings of others, and then convey this understanding with well-chosen words.

*Awareness of another person's feelings tends to cement friendships because the individual feels that "someone understands me."

Be a good listener.

There is a natural tendency to insinuate one's own opinions during conversation. A wise person enriches both the mind and the friendship by working hard at being a good listener, and not interrupting. However, this does not mean remaining silent. Shakespeare spoke of this matter in *Hamlet* when Polonius advised Laertes: "Give every man thine ear, but few thy voice."

Also try to understand EXACTLY what the speaker is saying, and where he or she is coming from. Careful listening is an art that can pay handsome dividends by reducing error and confusion. Cultivate it.

Ask questions appropriately and in a manner that does not appear to challenge or imply skepticism.

There are various aspects to this important communications skill. If a statement is not clear to you, set the record straight by asking, "Would you restate your views about… ?," or "Would you elaborate on the point about… ?"

Choose your words carefully.

Prudent persons tend to be cautious about the use and interpretation of their words. They realize that harm can be done by applying incorrect labels or inappropriate judgmental terms—e.g., "neurotic"; "antisocial"; "lazy"; "immoral."

Similarly, numerous hurtful words and inflammatory phrases tend to generate hostility. Examples are "stupid," "bad," "dumb," "immature" and "irresponsible." This is verbal abuse. The effects can be seen years later in disturbed adults who require professional help.

Another notorious verbal punisher is "should." When used reflexively by parents ("You *should* have known better"), spouses ("You *shouldn't* have done that if you really love me"), or even at one's self ("I *shouldn't* have made that mistake"), the results are bound to be damaging.

Avoid expressing dogmatic opinions until all the facts have been considered.

Defer criticism about complex problems involving politics, religion, economics and personal interrelations when definitive answers are impossible. The wise person will temper an opinion with a qualifying phrase which lacks dogmatism—e.g., "It would seem that… " or "Isn't it possible that… ?"

Learn assertiveness without damaging the relationship.

Living or working with others inevitably entails differences of opinion and a clash of wills. Different needs and values—intergenerational conflict; saving or spending; the decision to marry or to cohabitate; beginning a family soon or deferring it; expressing indignation to a relative or co-worker who insists upon smoking in one's presence—can create much misery and stress.

Deviant attitudes or behavior ought to be dealt with in a way that does not destroy the relationship through insensitive criticism or anger. Defining and evaluating the problem openly could obviate the intensity of differences. But it requires an honest disclosure of one's feelings and needs, a concerted effort to listen to the other person's feelings, and expressed willingness to decide on some mutually acceptable solution.

REGARD "HAPPINESS" REALISTICALLY

The "pursuit of happiness" is ingrained in the American ethic. A clear perception of what this term really means to the individual constitutes a major hallmark of maturity.

> In his book, *When All You've Ever Wanted Isn't Enough*, Rabbi Harold Kushner (1986) commented that mature happiness is not achieved through its "pursuit" (as worded in the Declaration of Independence) in terms of accumulating wealth, property, knowledge, and the constant self-centered search for fun. Rather, it generally comes as a byproduct of living a meaningful life.

Happiness has been variously defined as "success in the art of living" (Collwood 1974) and "the certainty of being needed" (Lande 1979). Abiding happiness, however, ought to be differentiated from experiencing a good mood or transient pleasure; it is not achieved by blindly pursuing fantasies.

Happiness is fostered through optimism, realistic expectations, and involvement in activities that generate and reinforce self-esteem and confidence. Happiness does not necessarily depend on a happy childhood, strong religious feelings, excellent health, or the extent of one's education or income.

The following encompass many of the components of happiness. Some will be discussed more fully:

- Count your blessings… and pause long enough daily to enjoy life's "small miracles."

204

- Be satisfied with your lot, especially when it represents a maximal effort. A British expression avers: "Enough is as good as a feast."

- Maintain a kind interaction with your family and other persons.

- Learn to accept your limitations. Do not attempt to achieve unrealistic goals.

- Resist the temptation to become a "Renaissance" man or woman by venturing too far from your primary field of experience and expertise.

- Enjoy your work to obtain a sense of personal competence and fulfillment.

- Maintain interest in the surrounding world through a "decently stocked mind."

- Change those situations that can be modified, and accept the rest by adopting a different relationship to them... regardless of age. Recall that Grandma Moses began painting when most in her cohort were dead. Similarly, ballet dancers and opera stars who are past their prime can be valuable teachers to others.

- Maintain a sense of humor as an effective skill for coping. Learn to laugh at your awkwardness and shortcomings because these happenings are experienced universally. *Proverbs* (17:22) asserts: "A merry heart doeth good like a medicine."

- Constantly anticipate or plan new experiences to avoid "getting into a rut." Be adaptable!

- Learn to take one day at a time. Partake of its beauty and grasp the opportunities it affords.

- Minimize perfectionism. Many gifted persons undermine their physical and mental health by seeking perfectionism in work and life style. Perfectionistic behavior is known to spawn stress, migraine, hypertension, and a host of other medical or nervous disorders considered to be epiphenomena of AD (Chapter 16).

- Learn to enjoy your own company. An important component of effective and resourceful living is the ability to live with one's self without experiencing undue loneliness. *Aloneness is not necessarily loneliness.* Ralph Waldo Emerson noted in *Self-Reliance:* "Nothing is at last sacred but the integrity of your own mind."

- Assist others on life's path, especially younger persons seeking a compassionate mentor with experience.

MINIMIZE "THE HURRY DISEASE"

"The hurry disease" exacts high physical, neurological and emotional tolls in a competitive society that rewards materialistic gain, business-professional achievement, and "upward mobility." It also has been referred to as "workaholism," "urgency addiction," and "Type A behavior."

Characteristics of this condition include rapid speech, fast eating, rapid moving, a proneness to frustration if one's pace is slowed (as in traffic), attempting to do several things simultaneously, the inability to forget business and professional concerns temporarily (even when on vacation), and guilt or anxiety evoked by relaxation. Other behavioral patterns include (1) a proneness to accept additional responsibility despite an existing heavy load and many demands on one's time, (2) being bored by a conversation that is not of active interest to the person, (3) a constant search for "more," and (4) few real hobbies.

The distinction should be made between a hard worker who sets realistic goals of work and rest, and the workaholic who cannot slow down. Dr. John L. Bulette (1979) described such an individual as "the person who is driven to achieve, who can't put time aside to develop any other gratifying areas of his or her life."

Drs. Meyer Friedman and Ray H. Rosenman (1974) pioneered the understanding of Type A behavior, especially as a contributory risk factor in coronary heart disease. (The latter is controversial, and some cardiologists disagree.) Germane to the present subject is neurotransmitter and metabolic dysfunction induced within the brain by workaholic habits and information overload. These changes can culminate in conditions such as migraine, depression, and "degenerative" diseases.

Type A behavior patterns became recognized more frequently among women when they increasingly entered demanding business and professional fields. For example, coronary heart disease quadrupled among "liberated" females in Japan (Friedman 1974). Also, such behavior can be transmitted to young children through constant parental urging about aggressive competitiveness, the primacy of achievement, and remaining in "the fast lane." (John Jensen aptly quipped: "The trouble with life in the fast lane is that you get to the other end in an awful hurry.")

Modifying Type A Behavior

Most persons with the hurry disease not only recognize such behavior, but also the threat of ruin that can result from the vicious cycle of excessively pursuing physical and psychological demands. The following constructive measures have benefitted many patients. They are modified adaptations of the recommendations by Drs. Friedman and Rosenman (1974) in *Type A Behavior and Your Heart*. Some were alluded to earlier.

- Live one day at a time. Sir William Osler underscored the importance of living in "day-tight compartments." A sentence from the Jewish Memorial Service *(Yizkor)* also is germane: "Teach us to number our days that we may get us a heart of wisdom." Another apt saying: "Live each day fully—as if it is the last one."

- Take time to give thanks for the blessings and opportunities that flow from the gift of life. The expression of such heartfelt gratitude, at whatever level, serves to brake the affliction of constant hurry.

- Always remember that most prior successes resulted from proper decisions and actions after careful thought in a relaxed—not hurried—mode. Often, mistakes can be attributed to hasty thinking and stereotyped action during "the rat race," especially when one is fatigued. As emphasized earlier, fatigue may be checked or minimized through rest periods, the avoidance of stimulants and other drugs (including alcohol), and by maintaining pleasant relationships with others.

- Set goals that are realistic… based on an honest evaluation of personal values and abilities. Special attention must be directed the "numbers game" (e.g., the number of clients or patients). Moreover, two sets of goals should be identified—accomplishments in one's business or professional career, and accomplishments in one's private life.

- <u>Attempt to make deadlines reasonable.</u> It has been quipped that persons with Type A behavior could benefit from monitoring deadlines with a calendar rather than a stopwatch.

- <u>Recognize and accept your personal limitations relative to ability, age, and other pertinent considerations.</u> In this respect, the standardized "average" individual should be regarded as a nonexistent mythical person.

- <u>Recognize and accept that your work is never truly finished, and act accordingly.</u> A workaholic ought to acknowledge this truism as it pertains to working late at night habitually, refusing to take breaks, and resisting vacations. Lin Yutang aptly observed: "Besides the noble art of getting things done, there is the noble art of leaving things undone."

- <u>Select a different vocabulary in order to change attitude and reduce self-imposed pressures.</u> An example is use of the expression "I choose to… "—rather than "I have to"—in matters such as chauffeuring children or doing volunteer work.

- <u>Anticipate boring delays by carrying pleasurable or inspirational reading material.</u> Persons with Type A behavior ought to welcome such "free time" for savoring enjoyable literature whose reading had been put off. For instance, being caught in a traffic jam, or waiting for a medical-dental appointment or a late-arriving friend, provides the opportunity for such reading time.

- <u>Develop work habits to contain the hurry disease.</u> Some examples:
  * Plan to arrive and leave in ways that minimize the frustration of traffic and rush-hour crowds.
  * Arrive at work early in order to clear your desk ("the art of deskmanship"), and to coordinate the day's activities.
  * Allow time for "catch up" periods and an unhurried lunch.
  * Delegate responsibility for handling trivia.
  * Avoid excessive conversations and unnecessarily prolonged visits.
  * Learn how to use the telephone efficiently.
  * Enjoy a few absorbing interests at a leisurely pace. A hobby is not truly recreational for an workaholic if it entails the sense of hurry or competition.

- <u>Strive for enlightened simplicity.</u> Seeking simplicity in conduct can serve as an antidote to the psychic drain that follows in the wake of excessive preoccupation with detail. This message was understood by great sages long before the computer era. A passage in the *Hallel* service perceptively states:

> "The Lord guardeth the simple;
> When I was brought low, he saved me."

- *Use vacations wisely.* Workaholics need vacations that represent a *true* departure from the routine. Near-total relaxation and integrated peace can be achieved by immersing oneself in a great book, listening intently to beautiful music, being uplifted by viewing nature's beauty, or by sharing joy in making love.

The ability to accept adversity and transform it to an advantage not only represents a great challenge, but also a major component for successful and healthy living. It is pertinent that the Chinese symbol for "crisis" means "opportunity" as well.

Failures and disappointments are inevitable, especially when goals are set too high (see above). But as in field sports, a person may not know his or her limits until they have been reached or exceeded. Learning how to respond appropriately and constructively to such setbacks is a notable achievement for reducing "destructive mind power."

Anticipate Responses to Problems.

One can develop the habit of confronting potential problems—financial, social or medical—by considering the appropriate responses in advance of action. The individual might reinforce them with a few basic attitudes, such as: "This, too, will pass," or "I have overcome even worse crises before." These behavioral patterns also help to build more confidence for coping with future difficulties.

Accept Reverses and Failure.

There is wisdom in recognizing that everyone makes mistakes. Unfortunately, the thought of failure erodes the mental peace of many persons because they view it not only as the loss of possessions and power, but also as rejection, humiliation, and depreciation of their worth. The associated anxiety then becomes an enormous drain of psychic energy. Walt Whitman focused on this matter in *Stronger Lessons:*

> "Have you not learned great lessons from those who reject you, and brace themselves against you? Or who treat you with contempt, or dispute the passage with you?"

This understandable attitude is usually inappropriate, especially for young people. If the individual is firmly committed to the belief that he or she can succeed, temporary reverses can enhance character through developing a sense of heightened determination and discipline.

> In his great essay, *Compensation*, Ralph Waldo Emerson noted the possible benefits of being confronted with adversity: "When he (man) is pushed, tormented, defeated, he puts on his wits, learns moderation and real skill... even the compensations of calamity are made apparent after long intervals of time."

Severe tension also results from confrontation with life-is-unfair situations, especially for persons who prided themselves on abiding by "the rules." Women face unique dilemmas in this sphere—e.g., an "empty nest"; early widowhood; desertion by a husband for a "younger model"; coping with a demented husband or parent. Under these circumstances, James Stockdale (1979) stated: "Life is unfair, but that does not justify you in acting unfairly."

"Change a Lemon Into a Lemonade."

We live in an era of considerable economic flux and instability. Many persons lose their job or personal security for reasons other than incompetence, and that are beyond their control. Yet, most of these reverses contain the seeds for overcoming them through optimism, redirecting skills and energies, "cooperating with the inevitable," and proper consultation.

- Mary Pickford asserted: "What we call failure is not the falling down, but the staying down."

- The attainment of ultimate success following disappointment and perceived defeat is illustrated by the despair of Nathaniel Hawthorne when he was dismissed from his government job. After listening to a tirade of complaints, his wife placed a pen and ink on the table, put her arms around him, and said: "Now you have the opportunity to write your novel." The result was *The Scarlet Letter.*

- Scores of my patients and friends have made "a lemonade from a lemon." Men who had a heart attack later confided: "Doctor, my attack was actually a blessing in disguise. It forced me to analyze my goals, and to channel my thinking and efforts in more fulfilling directions."

Attempt to Prevent the Peter Pan Syndrome in Children.

I have encountered the so-called Peter Pan syndrome (Chapter 13) in seemingly successful young persons and adults who were afflicted with severe anxiety, depression and loneliness. These features had culminated in considerable misery for themselves and their families. Dr. Dan Kiley (1983) subtitled his book on this disorder, *Men Who Have Never Grown Up.*

Such individuals tend to be the first children of affluent and permissive parents. Their intense anxiety commonly resulted from overemphasis upon perfectionism and the achievement of unrealistic goals.

The importance of preventing or minimizing this condition has become apparent both to mental health professionals and to seasoned parents—unfortunately often in retrospect. Many perplexed parents unsuccessfully sought the reason for a personality disorder of their oldest child until developing an awareness of the Peter Pan syndrome.

Kiley emphasized the need for parental self-examination aimed at correcting or reducing personal contributory traits.

- Fathers must reflect on their emotional life and behavior, such as engaging in self-pity, unwillingness to express their feelings, and giving a son covert messages about his mother's weakness.

- Mothers must recognize the elements of overprotectiveness and a patronizing attitude. Failure to insist upon responsible and consistent discipline by both the husband and the child tends to perpetuate the problems of inflexibility and self-centeredness.

- Both parents should really listen to one another, and attempt to communicate meaningfully, on these matters. This assumes much significance when a child is told that the other parent "shouldn't be bothered," or "doesn't understand personal feelings."

These insights are most valuable when a child under the age of 16 is not held accountable for his or her study habits and chores, and engages in excessive procrastination. It is important to impart "survival skills" for a son—including cooking, sewing, doing the laundry, and familiarity with tools. If such relationships and behavioral changes are ignored until the latter teens or adulthood, the Peter Pan syndrome (in the case of males) and the Cinderella complex (in the case of women who have retreated from responsibility) often require professional assistance to reduce future misery.

BIBLIOGRAPHY

Adamkiewicz, V.W.: Glycemia and immune responses. *Canadian Medical Association Journal* 1963; 88:806.

Adams, H.: *The Education of Henry Adams.* Boston, Massachusetts Historical Society, 1918.

Adolfsson, R., Bucht, G., Lithner, F., Winblad, D.: Hypoglycemia in Alzheimer's disease. *Acta Medica Scandinavica* 1980; 208:387-388.

Aeppel, T.: U.S. aluminum makers find world market a scary place. *The Wall Street Journal* 1993; November 8: B-4.

a. Agid, Y., et al: Differential vulnerability of cholinergic afferences to the mediodorsal thalamic nucleus in senile dementia of Alzheimer type and progressive supranuclear palsy. (Abstract) *Neurology* 1991; 41(Suppl.1):197.

b. Agid, Y., et al: Autoradiographic study of nerve growth factor receptor in the human forebrain of patients with Alzheimer's disease. *Neurology* 1991; 41(Suppl.1):199.

Allen, F.E.: One man's suffering spurs doctors to probe pesticide-drug link. *The Wall Street Journal* October 14, 1991, pp. A-1, A-4.

Anderson, K.K., Perez, G.L., Fisher, G.H., Man, E.H.: Effect of aluminum ingestion on aspartate racemization in the protein of rat brain. *Neuroscience Research Communications* 1990; 6:45-50.

Anderson, T.: Cited in *The Sciences.* November, 1973, p. 4.

Andrews, D.F. et al: Desferrioxamine for Alzheimer's disease. (Letter) *The Lancet* 1991; 338:325-326.

Angeletti, P.U., Liuzzi, A., Levi-Montalcini, R., Attardi, D.G.: Effect of a nerve growth factor on glucose metabolism by sympathetic and sensory nerve cells. *Biochemistry Biophysiology Acta* 1964; 90:445.

Angier, N.: How estrogen may work to protect against Alzheimer's. *The New York Times* 1994; March 8: B-6.

Alzheimer, A.: Über eine eigenartige Erkrankung der Hirnrinde. *Allgemeine Zeitschrift für Psychiatrie und Psychisch-Gerichtliche Medizin* 1907; 64:146-148.

Amiel, S.: Reversal of unawareness of hypoglycemia. *New England Journal of Medicine,* 1993; 329:876-877.

Antar, M.A., Ohlson, M.A., Hodges, R.E.: Changes in retail market food supplies in the United States in the last seventy years in relation to the incidence of essential fatty acids. *American Journal of Clinical Nutrition* 1964; 14:169.

Aono, J., Ueda, W., Manabe, M.: Alteration in glucose metabolism by crying in children. (Letter) *New England Journal of Medicine* 1993; 329:1129.

Arai, H., Schmidt, M.L., Lee, V., et al: Epitope analysis of senile plaque components in the hippocampus of patients with Parkinson's disease. *Neurology* 1992; 42:1315-1322.

Armon, C., Kurland, L.T., Daube, J.R., O'Brien, P.C.: Epidemiologic correlates of sporadic amyotrophic lateral sclerosis. *Neurology* 1991; 41:1077-1084.

Arregui, A., et al: High prevalence of migraine in high-altitude population. *Neurology* 1991; 41:1668-1670.

Arriagada, P.D., et al: Clinical-pathological correlations in Alzheimer's disease. (Abstract) *Neurology* 1991; 41(Suppl.1):407.

a. Arriagada, P., Growdon, J.H., Hedley-Whyte, E.T., Hyman, B.T.: Neurofibrillary tangles but not senile plaques parallel duration and severity of Alzheimer's disease. *Neurology* 1992; 42:631-639.

b. Arriagada, P.V., Marzloff, K., Hyman, B.T.: Distribution of Alzheimer-type pathologic changes in nondemented elderly individuals matches the pattern in Alzheimer's disease. *Neurology* 1992; 42:1681-1688.

Ashford, N.A., Miller, C.S.: *Chemical Sensitivity: A Report to the New Jersey State Department of Health.* December 1989.

Astrand, P.: Physical activity and fitness. *American Journal of Clinical Nutrition* 1992; 55(Suppl.6):1231-1236.

Bachman, D.L., Wolf, P.A., Linn, R., et al: Prevalence of dementia and probable senile dementia of the Alzheimer type in the Framingham Study. *Neurology* 1992; 42:115-119.

Baghurst, P.A., McMichael, A.J., Wigg, N.R., et al: Environmental exposure to lead and children's intelligences at the age of seven years: The Port Pirie Cohort Study. *New England Journal of Medicine* 1992; 327:1279-1284.

Banks, W.A., Kastin, A.J.: Aluminum increases permeability of the blood-brain barrier to labelled DSIP and β-endorphin: Possible implications for senile and dialysis dementia. *The Lancet* 1983; 322:1227-1229.

Banks, W.A., Kastin, A.J.: Aluminum-induced neurotoxicity: Alterations in membrane function at the blood-brain barrier. *Neuroscience & Biobehavioral Reviews* 1989; 13:47-53.

Barnes, D.N.: Neurotoxicity creates regulatory dilemma. *Science* 1989; 243:29-30.

Barnes, R.H., Neely, C.S., Kwong, E., Labandan, B.A., Frankova, S.: Postnatal nutritional deprivations as determinant of adult rat behavior toward food, its composition and utilization. *Journal of Nutrition* 1968; 96:90.

Barrett-Connor, E., Kritz-Silverstein, D.: Estrogen replacement therapy and cognitive function in older women. *Journal of the American Medical Association* 1993; 269:2637-2641.

Barrow, C.J., Zajorski, M.G.: Solution structures of ß peptide and its constituent fragments: Relation to amyloid deposition. *Science* 1991; 253:179-182.

Baulac, M., Lehericy, S., Chiras, J., et al: MR volumetric measurements of the hippocampal formation and amygdala in the mild stages of Alzheimer's disease. (Abstract) *Neurology* 1993; 43:A212.

Beral, V., Evans, S.: Malignant melanoma and exposure to fluorescent lighting at work. (Letter) *The Lancet* 1982; 319:1227.

Berger, A.R., Schaumburg, H.H., Schroeder, C., et al: Dose response, coasting, and differential fiber vulnerability in human toxic neuropathy: A prospective study of pyridoxine neurotoxicity. *Neurology* 1992; 42:1367-1370.

Beyreuther, K., Bush, A.R., Dyrks, T. et al: Mechanisms of amyloid deposition in Alzheimer's disease. In *Aging and Alzheimer's Disease*, edited by J. H. Glowdon, S. Corkin, E. Ritter-Walker and R. J. Wurtman, *Annals of the New York Academy of Sciences* 1991; 640:129-139.

Bishop, N., McGraw, M., Ward, N.: Aluminium in infant formulas. *The Lancet* 1989; 333:490.

Bixler, E.O., et al: Next-day memory impairment with triazolam use. *The Lancet* 1991; 337:827-831.

Bjorklund, G.: Mercury as a potential source for the etiology of Alzheimer's disease. *Trace Elements in Medicine* 1991; 8:208.

Bjorksten, J., Bjorksten, L., Nieto, D., Kleinstek, D.: Aluminum and neurofibrillary tangles as a cause of Alzheimer's disease; A hypothesis. *Journal of Advancement in Medicine* 1991; 4(Summer):121-130.

Blackman, J.D., Towle, B.L., Lewis, G.F., Spire, J., Polonsky, K.S.: Hypoglycemia thresholds for cognitive dysfunction in humans. *Diabetes* 1990; 39:828-835.

Blakeslee, S.: Mystery of sleep yields as studies reveal immune tie. *The New York Times* August 3, 1993, B-5, B-8.

Blanton, S.: The job your unconscious mind can do. In *How To Live With Life.* Reader's Digest Association, Inc., 1965, p.225.

Blass, J.P., Baker, A.C., Ko, L.: Alzheimer's disease: Inborn error of metabolism of late onset? In *Advances in Neurology, Volume 51: Alzheimer's Disease,* edited by R. J. Wurtman et al. Raven Press, Ltd., New York, 1990, pp.199-200.

Blass, J.P.: Pathophysiology of the Alzheimer's syndrome. *Neurology* 1993; 43(Suppl.4):S-25-38.

Boden, G., Chen, X., Desantis, R., et al: Effects of ethanol on carbohydrate metabolism in the elderly. *Diabetes* 1993; 42:28-34.

Borgaonkar, D.S., Schmidt, L.C., Martin, S.E., et al: Linkage of late-onset Alzheimer's disease with apolipoprotein E type 4 on chromosome 19. *The Lancet* 1993; 342:625.

Bornet, F.R.J., et al: Insulin and glycemic responses in healthy humans to native starches processed in different ways: Correlation with in vitro α-amylase hydrolysis. *American Journal of Clinical Nutrition* 1989; 50:315-323.

Bowen, A.J., Reeves, R.L.: Diurnal variation in glucose tolerance. *Archives of Internal Medicine* 1967; 119:261-264.

Bowen, D.M.: Treatment of Alzheimer's disease: Molecular pathology versus neurotransmitter-based therapy. *British Journal of Psychiatry* 1990; 157:327-330.

Bowmen, D.M., White, P., Spillane, J.A., et al: Accelerated aging or selective neuronal loss as an important cause of dementia? *The Lancet* 1979; 1:11-14.

Boyd, A.E., III, Lebovitz, H.E., Feldman, J.M.: Endocrine function and glucose metabolism in patients with Parkinson's disease and their alteration by L-dopa. *Journal of Clinical Endocrinology* 1971; 33:829-837.

212

Brayne, C., Calloway, D.: Normal ageing, impaired cognitive function, and senile dementia of the Alzheimer's type: a contiuum? *The Lancet* 1988; 1:1265-1266.

Breitner, J.C.S.: Clinical genetics and genetic counseling in Alzheimer's Disease. *Annals of Internal Medicine* 1991; 115:601-606.

Brenner, C., Merritt, H.H.: Effect of certain choline derivatives on the electrical activity of cortex. *Archives of Neurology and Psychiatry* 1942; 48;382.

Brenner, D.E., Kukull, W.A., van Belle, G. et al: Relationship between cigarette smoking and Alzheimer's disease in a population-based case-controlled study. (Abstract) *Neurology* 1992; 42:1322.

Brenner, S.: Aluminium, hot water tanks, and neurobiology. (Letter) *The Lancet* 1989; 333:781.

Brodan, V., et al: Influence of fructose on iron absorption from the digestive system of healthy subjects. *Nutrition Dieta* 1967; 9:263-270.

Brody, J.E.: Personal health. *The New York Times 1993*; June 16:B-7.

Brody, J.E.: Scientists measure the value of breast milk. *The New York Times* 1994; April 6: B-7.

Brown, R.G., Morrisden, C.D.: How common is dementia in Parkinson's disease? *The Lancet* 1984; II:1262-1265.

Brownlee, M., et al: Association of insulin pump therapy with raised serum amyloid A in type I diabetes mellitus. *The Lancet* 1984; 323:411-413.

Brownstein, N.J., Rehfeld, J.F.: Molecular forms of cholecystokinin in the nervous system. In *Neuronal Cholecystokinin*, edited by J. Vanderhaeghen and J. N. Crawley, *Annals of the New York Academy of Sciences* 1985; 448:9-10.

Brunner, E.A., Passonneau, J.V., Molstad, C.: The effect of volatile anesthetics on levels of metabolites and metabolic rate in brain. *Journal of Neurochemistry* 1971; 18:2301-2316.

Bryson, D.D.: Health hazards of formaldehyde. *The Lancet* 1981; 1:1263.

Bucht, G., et al: Changes in blood glucose and insulin secretion in patients with senile dememtia of Alzheimer's type. *Acta Medica Scandinarica* 1983; 213:387-392.

Buckwalter, J.G., Murdock, G.A., Miller, C.A., Henderson, V.W.: Gender-associated neuropathological features of Alzheimer's disease. (Abstract) *Neurology* 1993; 43:A251.

Buell, S.J., Coleman, P.D.: Dendritic growth in the aged human brain and failure of growth in senile dementia. *Science* 1979; 206:854-586.

Bush, A.: Cited in *Journal of the American Medical Association* 1994; 271:90.

Butler, P.C. Chou, J., Carter, W.B., et al: Effects of meal ingestion on plasma amylin concentration in NIDDM and nondiabetic humans. *Diabetes* 1990; 39:752-756.

Butterfield, W.J.H., Abrams, M.E., Sells, R.A., Sterky, G., Wichelow, H.J.: Insulin sensitivity of the human brain. *The Lancet* 1966; 1:557.

Butterworth, K.R., Drewitt, P.N., Springall, C.D., Morhouse, S.R.: Bioavailability of aluminium. (Letter) *The Lancet* 1992; 339;1489.

Caballero, B., Gleason, R.E., Wurtman, R.J.: Plasma amino acid concentrations in healthy elderly men and women. *American Journal of Clinical Nutrition* 1991; 53:1249-1252.

Callender, T.J.: Multiple chemical sensitivity syndrome and neurological abnormalities. Abstract, 26th Annual Meeting, American Academy of Environmental Medicine, Jacksonville, October 28, 1991, p. 19.

Campbell, N.R.C., Hasinoff, B.B., Stalts, H., et al: Ferrous sulfate reduces thyroxine efficacy in patients with hypothyroidism. *Annals of Internal Medicine* 1992; 117:1010-1013.

Candy, J.M., et al: Aluminosilicates and senile plaque formation in Alzheimer's Disease. *The Lancet* 1986; 327:354-356.

Caplan, J., Frederickson, P.A., Renaux, S.A., O'Brien, P.C.: Theophylline effect on sleep in normal subjects. *Chest* 1993; 103:193-195.

Caselli, R.J., Scheitajuer, B.W., O'Duffy, J.D., et al: Chronic inflammatory meningoencephalitis should not be mistaken for Alzheimer's disease. *Mayo Clinic Proceedings* 1993; 68:846-853.

Centers for Disease Control: Prevalence of chronic migranie headaches—United States, 1988-1989. *Morbidity and Mortality Weekly Report* 1991; May 24, 331-338.

Chandra, R.K.: Effect of vitamin and trace-element supplementation on immune responses and infection in elderly subjects. *The Lancet* 1992; 340:1124-1127.

Chang-Enger, M., Simko, A., Sosa, G., et al: Iron supplementation for premature infants with birthweight less than 1500 grams. *Clinical Research* 1993; 41:73A.

Chapman, A.G., Engelsen, B., Meldrum B.S.: 2-Amino-7-phosphonoheptanoic acid inhibits insulin-induced convulsions and striatal aspartate accumulation in rats with frontal cortical ablation. *Journal of Neurochemistry* 1987; 49:121-127.

Chen, Y.J., Guo, Y., Hsu, C., Rogan, W.J.: Cognitive development of Yu-Cheng ("oil disease") children prenatally exposed to heat-degraded PCBs. *Journal of the American Medical Association* 1992; 268:3213-3218.

Cheng, B., Mattson, M.P.: Glucose deprivation elicits neurofibrillary tangle-like antigenic changes in hippocampal neurons: Prevention by NGF and bFGF. *Experimental Neurology* 1992; 117:114-123.

Choi, D.W.: Anti-excitotoxic approaches to the treatment of hypoxic-ischemic neuronal injury. Invitational lecture, 43rd Annual Meeting, American Academy of Neurology, Boston, April 23, 1991.

Choi, D.W.: Bench to bedside: The glutamate connection. *Science* 1992; 258:241-243.

Choi, T.B., Yang, J., Pardridge, W.M.: Phenylalanine transport at the human-blood-brain barrier: Studies with isolated brain capillaries. *Diabetes* 1986; 35(Suppl.1):196.

Claus, J.J., van Harskamp, F., Breteler, M.M.B., et al: The diagnostic value of SPECT with Tc 99m HMPAO in Alzheimer's disease: A population-based study. *Neurology* 1994; 44:454-461.

Committee on Sciences and Technology, U.S. House of Representatives: *Neurotoxins: At Home And The Workplace.* Washington, U.S. Government Printing Office, 1989, Report 99-827.

Cook, M.: Cane fires nontoxic, farmers insist. *The Miami Herald* March 23, 1991, p.B-1.

Coon, J.J.: Food toxicology: Safety of food additives. *Modern Medicine* November 30, 1970, p.105.

Coon, P.J., Rogus, E.M., Drinkwater, D., et al: Role of body fat distribution in the decline in insulin sensitivity and glucose tolerance with age. *Journal of Clinical Endocrinology and Metabolism* 1992; 75:1125-1132.

Cooper, H.: Once again, ads woo teens with slang. *The Wall Street Journal* March 29, 1993, B-1.

Coren, S.: Left-handedness in offspring as a function of maternal age at parturition. (Letter) *New England Journal of Medicine* 1990; 322:1673.

Coriat, A.M., Gillard, R.D.: Beware the cups that cheer. (Letter) *Nature* 1986; 321:570.

Cornblath, M., Joassin, G., Weisskopf, B., Swiatek, K.R.: Hypoglycemia in the newborn. *Pediatric Clinics of North America* 1966; 13:905-920.

Corter, E.H., Saunders, A.M., Strittmatter, W.J., et al: Gene dose of apolipoprotein E type 4 allele and the risk of Alzheimer's disease in late onset families. *Science* 1993; 261:921-923.

Cottrell, J.J.: Altitude exposures during air craft flights; flying higher. *Chest* 1988; 93:81-84

Couratier, P., Sindou, P., Delacourte, A., et al: Abnormal βA4 amyloid immunostaining linked to glutamate toxicity. (Abstract) *Neurology* 1993; 43:A251.

Crapper, D.R., Krishnan, S.S., Quittkat, S.: Aluminium, neurofibrillary degeneration and Alzheimer's disease. *Brain* 1976; 99:67-80.

Crapper-McLachlan, D.R., et al: Intramuscular desferrioxamine in patients with Alzheimer's disease. *The Lancet* 1991; 337:1304-1308.

Cravioto, J., Robles, B.: Evolution of adaptive and motor behavior during rehabilitation for kwashiorkor, *American Journal of Orthopsychiatry* 1965; 35:499-502.

Crawley, J.N.: Comparative distribution of cholecystokinin and other neuropeptides. In *Neuronal Cholecystokinin*, edited by J. Vanderhaeghen and J. N. Crawley, *Annals of the New York Academy of Sciences* 1985; 448:1-8.

Crosby, W.H.: Dietary iron overload. *New England Journal of Medicine* 1992; 326:1705.

Cross, A.J., Slater, D., Simpson, M., et al: Sodium dependent D-(3H) aspartate binding in cerebral cortex in patients with Alzheimer's and Parkinson's diseases. *Neurosciences Letter* 1987; 79:213-217.

214

Culter, N.R., et al: Brain metabolism as measured with positron emission tomography: Serial assessment in a patient with familial Alzheimer's disease. *Neurology* 1985; 35:1556-1561.

Cutler, P.: Deferoxamine therapy in high-ferritin diabetes. *Diabetes* 1989; 38:1207-1210.

Cutter, E.: Address on dietetics—medical food ethics now and to come. *Journal of the American Medical Association* 1893; 20:239-244.

Dart, B.: All the globe groaning from job-related stress. *The Palm Beach Post* March 23, 1993, A-1, A-7.

Dartigues, J.F., et al: Occupation during life and memory performance in the elderly: Results of the Paquid program. (Abstract) *Neurology* 1991; 41(Suppl.1):322.

Dartigues, J.F., Gagnon, M., Mazaux, J.M., et al: Occupation during life and memory performance in nondemented French elderly community residents. *Neurology* 1992; 42:1697-1701.

Davenport, A., Goodall, R.: Aluminum and dementia. (Letter) *The Lancet* 1992; 339:1236.

Davis, E.S.: Chemicals, risk and the public. *Chicago Tribune* 1989; April 29.

Davis, N.R., Shamoon, H.: Counterregulatory adaptation to recurrent hypoglycemia in normal humans. *Journal of Clinical Endocrinology and Metabolism* 1991; 73:995-1001.

Day, J.P., et al: Aluminium absorption study by ^{26}Al tracer. *The Lancet* 1991; 337:1345.

de Leon, M.J., Golomb, G.J., Covit, A., et al: Hippocampal formation atrophy: A biological marker predicting Alzheimer's disease. (Abstract) *Neurology* 1993; 43;A405.

a. Deveny, K.: Wine contains too much lead, government tests find. *The Wall Street Journal* 1991; June 6: B-1.

b. Deveny, K.: Wine makers criticize study showing high levels of lead in their products. *The Wall Street Journal* 1991; August 2: p. B-8.

Diamond, M.P., et al: Suppression of counterregulatory hormone response to hypoglycemia by insulin per se. *Journal of Clinical Endocrinology and Metabolism* 1991; 72:1388-1390.

Dillard, T.A., Beninati, W.A., Berg, B.W.: Air travel in patients with chronic obstructive pulmonary disease. *Archives of Internal Medicine* 1991; 151:1793-1795.

Domingo, J.L., Gomez, M., Llobet, J.M., Richart, C.: Effect of ascorbic acid on gastrointestinal aluminium absorption. *The Lancet* 1991; 338:1467.

Duara, R., Lopez-Alberola, R.F., Barker, W.W., et al: A comparison of familial and sporadic Alzheimer's disease. *Neurology* 1993; 43:1377-1384.

Duffy, J.: Eosinophilia-myalgia syndrome. *Mayo Clinic Proceedings* 1992; 67:1201-1202.

Duggan, J.: Cited by *Medical Tribune* 1992; July 23: C-1.

During, M.J., Spencer, D.D.: Extracellular hippocampal glutamate and spontaneous seizure in the conscious human brain. *The Lancet* 1993; 341:1607-1610.

Edwardson, J.A., Moore, P.B., Ferrier, I.N., et al: Effect of silicon on gastrointestinal absorption of aluminium. *The Lancet* 1993; 342:211-212.

Elliott, K.A.C., Page, I.H., Quastel, J.H.: *Neurochemistry.* Charles C Thomas, Springfield, 1962.

Fairechild, D.: *Jet Smart.* Flyana Rhyme, Inc., Maui, 1993.

Feldberg, W.: Present views on the mode of action of acetylcholine in the central nervous system. *Physiology Reviews* 1945; 25:596.

Felton, J.: Cited by *The Miami Herald* 1991; April 24: D-2.

Fennell, E.D., Booth, M.P., Moberg, P.J., Gallagher, T.J.: Neuropsychological evaluation of 13 cases of acute simultaneous exposure to moderate levels of carbon monoxide. (Abstract) *Neurology* 1991; 41(Suppl.1):237.

Ferrari, M.D., et al: Neuroexcitatory plasma amino acids are elevated in migraine. *Neurology* 1990; 40:1582-1586.

Fioravanti, M., et al: Relationship between hypertension and early indicators of cognitive decline. *Dementia* 1991; 2:51-56.

Fischer, W., et al: Amelioration of cholinergic neuronal atrophy and spacial memory impairment in aged rats by nerve growth factor. *Nature* 1987; 329:65-68.

Fisher, C.E., Knowles, M.E., Massey, R.C., McWeeny, D.J.: Levels of aluminium in infant formulae. *The Lancet* 1989; 333:1024.

Floyd, J.C., Jr., Fajans, S., Conn, J.W., Knopf, R.F., Rull, J.: Stimulation of insulin secretion by amino acids. *Journal of Clinical Investigation* 1966; 45:1487-1502.

Floyd, J.C., Fajans, S., Pek, S., et al: Synergistic effect of certain amino acid pairs upon insulin secretion in man. *Diabetes* 1970; 19:102-108.

Forbes, W.F., Hayward, L.M., Agwani, N.: Dementia, aluminium, and fluoride. *The Lancet* 1991; 338:1592-1593.

Forbes, W.F., McAniey, C.A.: Aluminium and dementia. (Letter) *The Lancet* 1992; 340:668-669.

Frank, R.E., Serdula, M.K., Adame, D.: Weight loss and bulimic eating behavior: Changing patterns within a population of young adult women. *Southern Medical Journal* 1991; 84:457-460.

Frasure-Smith, N., Lespérance, F., Talajic, M.: Depression following myocardial infarction: Impact on 6-month survival. *Journal of the American Medical Association* 1993; 270:1819-1925.

Frazier, W.A., Hogue-Angeletti, R.A., Bradshaw, R.A.: Nerve growth factor versus insulin. (Letter) *Science* 1973; 180:1301-1302.

Friedland, R.P., et al: Alzheimer disease: Clinical and biological heterogeneity. *Annals of Internal Medicine* 1988; 109:298-311.

Friedman, J.H., Levy, H.L., Boustany, R.M.: Late onset of distinct neurologic syndromes in galactosemic siblings. *Neurology* 1989; 39:741-742.

Friedman, M., Rosenman, R.H.: *Type A Behavior and Your Heart* Alfred A. Knopf, Inc., New York, 1974.

Froede, H.C., Wilson, I.B.: The slow rate of inhibition of acetylcholinesterase by fluoride. *Molecular Pharmacology* 1985; 27:630-633.

Fudenberg, H.H.: Cited by *The Last Chance Health Report* 1993; 3 (#4):1-8.

Fujisawa, Y., Sasaki, K., Akijama, K.: Increased insulin levels after 06TT load in perifheral blood and cerebrospinal fluid of patients with dementia of Alzheimer's type. *Biological Psychiatry* 1991; 30:1219-1228.

Fuller, C.J., Faulkner, H., Bendich, A., et al: Effect of β-carotene supplementation on photosuppression of delayed-type hypersensitivity in normal young men. *American Journal of Clinical Nutrition* 1992; 56;684-690.

Garruto, R.M., et al: Imaging of calcium and aluminum in neurofibrillary tangle bearing neurons in Parkinsonism-dementia of Guam. *Proceedings of the National Academy of Sciences U.S.A.* 1984; 81:1875.

Garry, P.J., Wayne, S.J., Koehler, K.M., et al: Prediction of iron absorption based on iron status of female blood donors. *American Journal of Clinical Nutrition* 1992; 56:691-698.

Gilley, D.W., et al: Cessation of driving and unsafe motor vehicle operation by dementia patients. *Archives of Internal Medicine* 1991; 151:941-946.

Giugliano, D., Salvatore, T., Cozzolino, D., et al: Hyperglycemia and obesity as determinants of glucose, insulin, and glucagon responses to β-endorphin in human diabetes mellitus. *Journal of Clinical Endocrinology and Metabolism* 1987; 64:1122-1128.

Goldsmith, J.R., Landaw, S.A.: Carbon monoxide and human health. *Science* 1968; 162:1352.

Goleman, D.: A rising cost of modernity: Depression. *The New York Times* 1992; December 8:C-1, C-13.

Goleman, D.: Mental decline in aging need not be inevitable. *The New York Times* 1994; April 26:B-5.

Goltermann, N.R.: The biosynthesis of cholecystokinin in neural tissue. In *Neuronal Cholecystokinin,* edited by J. Vanderhaeghen and J. N. Crawley, *Annals of the New York Academy of Sciences* 1985; 448:76-86.

Gomez, B., Garcia-Villallon, A.L., Frank, A., et al: Effects of hypoglycemia on the cerebral circulation in awake goats. *Neurology* 1992; 42:909-916.

Good, R.A.: Cited in *Internal Medicine News & Cardiology News* 1993; October 1: 6.

Gordon, G.S. Elliott, H.W.: Action of diethylstilbestrol and some steroids on respiration of rat brain homogenates. *Endocrinology* 1947; 41:517.

Gorell, J.M., Brienza, R.S., Johnson, C.C.: Metal exposure and Parkinson's disease mortality. (Abstract) *Neurology* 1991; 41(Suppl.1):308.

Graves, A.B., White, E., Koepsell, T.D., et al: The association between aluminum-containing products and Alzheimer's disease. *Journal of Clinical Epidemiology* 1990; 43:35-44.

Greenough, W.T., Green, E.J.: Experience and the changing brain. In *Aging, Biology, and Behavior,* edited by J. McGaugh and S. Kiesler. Academic Press, New York 1981:159-193.

Gross, K.C., Acosta, P.B.: Fruits and vegetables are a source of galactose: Implications in planning the diets of patients with galactosemia. *Journal of Inherited Metabolic Diseases* 1991; 14:253:258.

Growdon, J.H.: Treatment for Alzheimer's disease? *New England Journal of Medicine* 1992; 327:1306-1308.

Gutfeld, R.: Lead in water of many cities is found excessive. *The Wall Street Journal* October 21, 1992, p. B-7.

Hachinski, V.: Preventable senility: A call for action against the vascular dementias. *The Lancet* 1992; 340:645-648.

Hack, M., et al: Effect of very low birth weight and subnormal head size on cognitive abilities at school age. *New England Journal of Medicine* 1991; 325:231-237.

Haier, R.J.: Cerebral glucose correlates of personality and intelligence. Presented at annual meeting of the American Association for the Advancement of Science, Boston, February 14, 1988.

Hallfrisch, J.: Fructose and blood cholesterol. *American Journal of Clinical Nutrition* 1993; 57:89.

Halpern, D.F., Coren, S.: Handedness and life span. *New England Journal of Medicine* 1991; 324:998.

Hammond, E.C.: Factors in the etiology of coronary heart disease, stroke and aortic aneurysm. Presented at Albany Medical College, Albany, New York, October 17, 1968.

Hampson, N.B., Kramer, C.C., Copass, M.K.: Unintentional carbon monoxide poisoning following winter storm—Washington, January 1993. *Journal of the American Medical Association* 1993; 269:1372-1373.

Hampson, N.B., Kramer, C.C., Gunford, R.G., Norkool, D.M.: Carbon monoxide poisoning from indoor burning of charcoal briquets. *Journal of the American Medical Association* 1994: 271:52-53.

Harik, S.I., Kalaria, R.N.: Blood-brain barrier abnormalities in Alzheimer's disease. In *Aging and Alzheimer's Disease,* edited by J. H. Growdon, S. Corkin, E. Ritter-Walker and R. J. Wurtman, *Annals of the New York Academy of Sciences* 1991; 640:47-52.

Harrell, L.E., Davis, J.M.: Cholinergic influences on hippocampal glucose metabolism. *Neuroscience* 1985; 15:359-369.

Harrigan, M.R., Malouf, A.T.: The effect of beta-amyloid on rat hippocampal slice cultures. *Clinical Research* 1993; 41:3A.

Harris, D.N.F., Bailey, S.M., Smith, P.L.C., et al: Brain swelling in first hour after coronary artery bypass surgery. *The Lancet* 1993; 342:586-587.

Haworth, J.C., McRae, K,N.: The neurological development effects of neonatal hypoglycemia: A follow-up of 22 cases. *Canadian Medical Association Journal* 1965; 92:861-865.

Hayden, D., Siminoski, K.: In vivo regulation of tissue nerve growth factor levels by thyroid hormone. Abstract 976. 74th Annual Meeting of the Endocrine Society, San Antonio, June 24, 1992.

Heaton, K.W., Marcus, S.N., Emmett, P.M., Bolton, C.H.: Particle size of wheat, maize, and oat test meals: Effects on plasma glucose and insulin responses and on the rate of starch digestion in vitro. *American Journal of Clinical Nutrition* 1988; 47:675-682.

Hendee, W.R.: There's no free lunch: The benefits and risks of technologies. *Journal of the American Medical Association* 1991; 265:1437-1438.

Henderson, A.S.: Epidemiology of dementia disorders. In *Advances in Neurology. Volume 51: Alzheimer's Disease,* edited by R. J. Wurtman et al. Raven Press, Ltd., New York, 1990, pp.15-25.

Hersey, P., Hasic, E., Edwards, A., et al: Immunological effect of solarium exposure. *The Lancet* 1983; 1:545-548.

Heyman, A., et al: Alzheimer's disease: A study of epidemiological aspects. *Annals of Neurology* 1984; 15:335-341.

Hodges, R.E., Krehl, W.A.: The role of carbohydrates in lipid metabolism. *American Journal of Clinical Nutrition* 1965; 17:334.

Hoeldtke, R.D., Boden, G.: Epinephrine secretion, hypoglycemia unawareness, and diabetic autonomic neuropathy. *Annals of Internal Medicine* 1994; 120:512-517.

Hoffman, A.: The epidemiology of Alzheimer's disease. (Abstract) *Neuroepidemiology* 1991; 10:101.

Holbrook, J.T., Smith, J.C., Jr., Reiser, S.: Dietary fructose or starch: Effects on copper, zinc, iron, manganese, calcium and magnesium balances in humans. *American Journal of Clinical Nutrition* 1989; 49:1290-1294.

Holmes, C.S.: Cognitive functioning and diabetes: Broadening the paradigm for behavioral and health psychology? *Diabetes Care* 1987; 10:135-136.

Holmes, O.W.: Cited by the *Journal of the American Medical Association* 1892; June 18.

Honigman, B., Theis, M.K., Koziol-McLain, J., et al: Acute mountain sickness in general tourist population at moderate altitudes. *Annals of Internal Medicine* 1993; 118:587-592.

Hoover, J.: Ice cream: A chemical nightmare. *Townsend Letter for Doctors* 1993; April: 376.

Hornbein, T.F., Townes, B.D., Schoene, R.B., et al: The cost to the central nervous system of climbing to extremely high altitude. *New England Journal of Medicine* 1989; 321:1714-1719.

Hoyer, S., Oesterreich, K., Wagner, O.: Glucose metabolism as the site of the primary abnormality in early-onset dementia of Alzheimer type? *Journal of Neurology* 1988; 235:143-148.

Hoyer, S.: Abnormalities of glucose metabolism in Alzheimer's disease. In *Aging and Alzheimer's Disease,* edited by J. H. Growdon, S. Corkin, E. Ritter-Walker and R. J. Wurtman, *Annals of the New York Academy of Sciences* 1991; 640:53-58.

Hoyer, S.: Abnormalities in brain glucose utilization and its impact on cellular and molecular mechanisms in sporadic dementia of Alzheimer type. In *Alzheimer's Disease,* edited by R. M. Nitsch, J. H. Growdon, S. Corkin, R. J. Wurtman. *Annals of the New York Academy of Sciences* 1993; 695:77-80.

Hruska, R.E., Chertack, M.M., Kravis, D.: Elevation of nerve growth factor receptor-truncated in the urine of patients with diabetic neuropathy. *Annals of the New York Academy of Sciences* 1993; 679:349-351.

Hunter, B.T.: Some nutritional shortchanging from food processing. *Journal of the International Academy of Preventive Medicine* 1977; Winter:59-71.

Hunter, B.T.: Health risks from some methods of preparing foods. *Clinical Ecology* 1984:3; 189-194.

a. Hunter, B.T.: Food health claims: Fact vs fiction. *Consumers' Research* May 1991, p. 13.

b. Hunter, B.T.: Some health risks from innovative packaging and processing practices. Presented at Annual Meeting, American Academy of Environmental Medicine, Jacksonville, October 29, 1991.

Hunter, B.T.: Some unanticipated interactions. *Consumer's Research* 1993; December: 8-9.

Husband, A.J.: *Psychoimmunology: CNS Immune Interactions.* CRC Press, Inc., Boca Raton (Florida), 1993.

a. Hyman, B.T.: Hippocampal anatomy and Alzheimer's disease. *Neurochemistry.* Course Number 340, American Academy of Neurology, Boston, April 26, 1991.

b. Hyman, B.T., Mann, B.M.A.: Neurofibrillary pathology in Down's syndrome in individuals of various age. In *Alzheimer's Disease: Basic Mechanisms, Diagnosis and Therapeutic Strategy,* edited by K. Iqbal, B. R. C. McLachlan, B. Windlad, and H. M. Wisniewski. Wiley, 1991, pp.105-115.

Im, H.S., Barnes, R.H., Levitzky, D.A.: Postnatal malnutrition and brain cholinesterase in rats. *Nature* 1971; 233:269-270.

Isaacson, R.: Cited in *The Wall Street Journal* 1992; October 28: B-6.

Jack, C.R., Jr., Petersen, R.C., O'Brien, P.C., Tangalos, E.G.: MR-based hippocampal volumetry in the diagnosis of Alzheimer's disease. *Neurology* 1992; 42:183-188.

Jackson, B.T., Cohn, H.E., Morrison, S.H., et al: Hypoxia-induced sympathetic inhibition of the fetal plasma insulin response to hyperglycemia. *Diabetes* 1993; 42:1621-1625.

Jackson, J.A., Riordan, H.D., Poling, C.N.: Aluminum from a coffee pot. *The Lancet* 1989; 1:781-782.

Jaouni, S., Allmann, D.W.: Effect of sodium fluoride and aluminum on cAMP, adenylate cyclase and phospho-diesterase activity. *Journal of Dental Research* 1985; 64:201.

Jarrett, R.J., Keen, H.: Diurnal variation of oral glucose tolerance: A possible pointer to the evolution of diabetes mellitus. *British Medical Journal* 1969; 2:341-343.

Jenkins, R., Hunt, S.P.: Long-term increase in levels of c-jun mRNA and jun protein-like immunoreactivity in motor and sensory neurons following axon damage. *Neuroscience Letters* 1991; 129:107-110.

Jeret, J.S., Mandell, M., Avitable, M.J.: "Mild" head trauma: A deceptive term. (Abstract) *Neurology* 1993; 43:A218.

Jobst, K.A., Smith, A.D. Szatmari, M., et al: Rapidly progressing atrophy of medial temporal lobe in Alzheimer's disease. *The Lancet* 1994; 343:829-830.

218

Jones, K.F., Berg, J.H.: Fluoride supplementation: A survey of pediatricians and pediatric dentists. *American Journal of Diseases of Children* 1992; 146:1488-1491.

Jones, T.W., et al: Mild hypoglycemia and impairment of brain stem and cortical evoked potential in healthy subjects. *Diabetes* 1990; 39:1550-1555.

Joosten, E., van den Berg, A., Riezler, R., et al: Metabolic evidence that deficiencies of vitamin B-12 (cobalamin), folate, and vitamin B-6 occur commonly in elderly people. *American Journal of Clinical Nutrition* 1993; 58:468-476.

Kahana, E., Gelper, Y., Korczyn, A.D.: Epidemiology of senile dementia: Protective effect of education. (Abstract) *Neurology* 1993; 43:A318.

Kalaria, R.N., Harik, S.I.: Reduced glucose transporter at the blood-brain barrier and in cerebral cortex in Alzheimer's disease. *Journal of Neurochemistry* 1989; 53:1083-1088.

Kalckar, H.M.: Galactose metabolism and cell "sociology." *Science* 1965; 150:305-312.

Karjalainen, J., Martin, J.M., Knip, M., et al: A bovine albumin peptide as a possible trigger of insulin-dependent diabetes mellitus. *New England Journal of Medicine* 1992; 327:302-307.

Kennedy, A.M., Newman, S.N., Warrington, E.K., et al: Familial Alzheimer's disease versus sporadic Alzheimer's disease: A clinical, neuropsychological and PET study. (Abstract) *Neurology* 1993; 43:A192.

Kenney, R.A., Tidball, C.S.: Human susceptibility to oral monosodium L-glutamate. *American Journal of Clinical Nutrition* 1972; 25:140-146.

Kerwin, J., et al: Distribution of nerve growth factor receptor immunoreactivity in the human hippocampus. *Neuroscience Letters* 1991; 121:178-182.

Kesslak, J.P., Nalcioglu, O., Cotman, C.W.: Quantification of magnetic resonance scans for hippocampal and parahippocampal atrophy in Alzheimer's disease. *Neurology* 1991; 41:51-54.

Kessler, D.: Cited by *The Palm Beach Post* 1993; June 15: A-7.

Khachaturian, Z.S.: New challenges in Alzheimer's disease and dementia research. In *Familial Alzheimer's Disease,* edited by G. D. Miner et al. Marcel Dekker, Inc., New York, 1989, pp.369-375.

Kiley, D.: *The Peter Pan Syndrome.* Dodd, Mead & Company, New York, 1993.

Kisters, K., et al: Aluminum concentrations and localization in gastric mucous membrane before and after therapy with aluminum containing antacids. *Trace Elements in Medicine* 1990; 7:199-202.

Klachko, D.M., Lie, T.H., Burns, T.W., Browne, J., Whitaker, J.: The effect of exercise on blood glucose levels of diabetics receiving insulin. *Clinical Research* 1968; 16:466.

Klein, T.W.: Stress and infection. *Journal of the Florida Medical Association* 1993; 80:409-411.

Klunk, W.E., et al: N-acetyl-L-aspartate, a neuronal marker detectable by NMR, decreases with progression of Alzheimer's disease. (Abstract) *Neurology* 1991; 41(Suppl.1):270.

Klunk, W.E., Panchalingam, K., Moossy, J., et al: N-acetyl-L-aspartate and other amino acid metabolites in Alzheimer's disease brain: A preliminary proton nuclear magnetic resonance study. *Neurology* 1992; 42:1578-1585.

Kokmen, E., et al: Prevalence of medically diagnosed dementia in a defined United States population: Rochester, Minnesota, January 1, 1975. *Neurology* 1989; 39:773-776.

Kokmen, E., et al: Clinical risk factors for Alzheimer's disease: A population-based case-control study. *Neurology* 1991; 41:1393-1397.

a. Kokmen, E., Beard, C.M., O'Brien, P.C., Kurland, L.T.: Educational attainment in Alzheimer's disease: Reassessment of the Rochester, Minnesota, data (1975-1984). (Abstract) *Neurology* 1993; 43:A316.

b. Kokmen, E., Beard, C.M., O'Brien, P.C., et al: Is the incidence of dementing illness changing? A 25-year time trend study in Rochester, Minnesota (1960-1984). *Neurology* 1993; 43:1887-1892.

Koller, W.C.: When does Parkinson's disease begin? *Neurology* 1992; 42(Suppl.4):27-31.

Kral, V.A., Emery, O.B.: Long-term follow-up of depressive pseudomentia of the aged. *Canadian Journal of Psychiatry* 1989; 34:445-446.

Krempf, M., Hoerr, R.A., Pelletier, V.A., et al: An isotopic study of the effect of dietary carbohydrate on the metabolic fate of dietary leucine and phenylalanine. *American Journal of Clinical Nutrition* 1993; 57:161-169.

Krupnick, A.J., Portney, P.R.: Controlling urban air pollution: A benefit-cost assessment. *Science* 1991; 252:522-528.

Kuhn, T.S.: *The Structure of Scientific Revolutions.* 2nd Edition, University of Chicago Press, Chicago, 1970.

Kumagae, Y., Matsui, Y.: Output, tissue levels, and synthesis of acetylcholine during and after transient forebrain ischemia in the rat. *Journal of Neurochemistry* 1991; 56:1169-1173.

Kushner, H.: *When All You've Ever Wanted Isn't Enough.* Kushner Enterprises, Inc. 1986.

Laedtke, T.W., Petersen, R.C., O'Brien, T.D., et al: Are Alzheimer's disease (AD) and non-insulin dependent diabetes (NIDDM) related? *Clinical Research* 1994; 42:65A.

Lagemann, J.K.: Forgiveness: The saving grace. In *How To Live With Life.* Reader's Digest Association, Inc., 1965, p. 469.

Lajtha, A.: The "brain barrier system." In *Neurochemistry,* edited by K. A. C. Elliott, I. H. Page, and J. H. Quastel. Charles C Thomas, Springfield, 1962, p. 410.

Lambert, A.E., Hoet, J.J.: Diurnal pattern of plasma insulin concentration in the human. *Diabetologia* 1966; 2:69.

Lande, L.M.: Personal communication, 1979.

Langston, J.W.: Parkinson's disease: The next decade of research. Address to the 43rd annual meeting of the American Academy of Neurology, Boston, April 24, 1991.

Lee, J.: Gilbert's disease and fluoride intake. *Fluoride* 1983; 16:139-145.

Lee, J.C.: The effects of alcohol injections on the blood-brain barrier. *Quarterly Journal of Studies on Alcohol* 1962; 23:4-16.

Lee, L.: *Radiation Protection Manual* 3rd Edition. Grassroots Network, Redwood City, 1990:107.

Li, G., Shen, Y.C., Li, Y.T., et al: A case-control study of Alzheimer's disease in China. *Neurology* 1992; 42: 1481-1488.

Lindenbaum, J., Rosenberg, I.H., Wilson, P.W.F., et al: Prevalence of cobalamin deficiency in the Framingham elderly population. *American Journal of Clinical Nutrition* 1994; 60:2-11.

Lipman, J.J., Colowick, S.P., Lawrence, P.L., Abumrad, N.N.: Aluminum induced encephalopathy in the rat. *Life Sciences* 1988; 42:863-875.

a. Lipman, J.J.: Cited in *The Psychiatric Times,* 1989; March: 11.

b. Lipman, J.J., Tolchard, S.: Comparison of the effects of central and peripheral aluminum administration on regional 2-deoxy-D-glucose in cooperation in the rat brain. *Life Sciences* 1989; 45:1977-1987.

Lipscomb, B.: Cited by the *Palm Beach Post* 1991; October 18:B-1.

Lipton, S.A., Rosenberg, P.A.: Excitatory amino acids as a final common pathway for neurologic disorders. *New England Journal of Medicine* 1994; 330:613-622.

Lorand, A.: *Old Age Deferred.* F. A. Davis Company, Philadelphia, 1910.

Lorscheider, F.L., Vimy, M.J.: Mercury exposure from "silver" fillings. *The Lancet* 1991; 337-1103.

Lou, J., Jankovic, J.: Essential tremor: Clinical correlates in 350 patients. *Neurology* 1991; 41:234-238.

Lubec, G., Wolf, C., Bartosch, B.: Amino acid isomerization and microwave exposure. *The Lancet* 1989; 2:1392-1393.

Lucas, A., Morley, R., Cole, T.J., et al: Breast milk and subsequent intelligence quotient in children born preterm. *The Lancet* 1992; 339:261-264.

Lukiw, W.J., Kruck, T.P.A., Crapper McLachlan, D.R.: Aluminium and the nucleus of nerve cells. *The Lancet* 1989; 333:781.

Mahler, M.E., et al: Glucose PET in dementia: DAT and MID compared. *Neurology* 1991; 41(Suppl.1):119.

Man, E.H., Sandhouser, M.E., Burg, J., Fisher, G.H.: Accumulation of D-aspartic acid with age in the human brain. *Science* 1983; 220:1407-1408.

a. Man, E.H., Bada, J.L.: Dietary D-amino acids. *Annual Review of Nutrition* 1987; 7:209-225.

b. Man, E.H., et al: D-aspartate in human brain. *Journal of Neurochemistry* 1987; 48:510-515.

Manson, J.E., Nathan, D.M., Krolewski, A.S., et al: A prospective study of exercise and incidence of diabetes among U.S. male physicians. *Journal of the American Medical Association* 1992; 268:63-67.

Marder, K., Tang, M., Cote, L., et al: Risk factors for dementia in Parkinson's disease. (Abstract) *Neurology* 1993; 43:A285.

Mark, V.H., Mark, J.P.: *Reversing Memory Loss.* Houghton Mifflin Company, New York, 1992.

Markowitz, S.B., Nunez, C.M., Klitzman, S., et al: Lead poisoning due to *hai ge fen*. *Journal of the American Medical Association* 1994; 271:932-934.

Marsden, C.D.: Parkinson's disease. *The Lancet* 1990; 335:948-952.

Martinez-Lage, J.M., Manubens, J.M., Lacruz, R., et al: Risk factors for Alzheimer's disease: A case-control study in Pamplona. (Abstract) *Neurology* 1992; 42(Suppl.3):141.

Martyn, C.N., Osmond, C., Edwardson, J.A., et al: Geographical relation between Alzheimer's disease and aluminium in drinking water. *The Lancet* 1989; 333:59-62.

Marx, J.: New clue found to Alzheimer's. *Science* 1991; 253:857-858.

Marx, J.: Alzheimer's debate boils over. *Science* 1992; 257:1336-1338.

Matsumoto, Y., Uyama, O., Shimizu, S., et al: Do anger and aggression affect carotid atherosclerosis? *Stroke* 1993; 24:983-986.

Mattson, M.P., Rydel,R.E., Lieberburg, R., Smith-Swintosky, V.L.: Altered calcium signaling and neuronal injury: Stroke and Alzheimer's disease as examples. In *Markers of Neuronal Injury and Degeneration,* edited by J. N. Johannessen, *Annals of the New York Academy of Sciences* 1993; 679:1-21.

May, D.S., et al: Surveillance of major causes of hospitalization among the elderly, 1988. *CDC Surveillance Summaries* 1991; 40:7-21.

Mayberg, H.S., Starkstein, S.E., Jeffery, P.J., et al: Limbic cortex hypometabolism in depression: Similarities among patients with primary and secondary mood disorders. (Abstract) *Neurology* 1992; 42(Suppl.3):181.

Max, W.: The economic impact of Alzheimer's disease. *Neurology* 1993; 43(Suppl.4):S-6-10.

McDougal, D.R., Jr., Schuls, D.W., Passonneau, J.V., et al: Quantitative studies of white matter. I. Enzymes involved in glucose-6-phosphate metabolism. *Journal of General Physiology* 1961; 44:487.

McDougal, D.B., Jr., Schimke, R.T., Jones, E.M., Touhill, E: Quantitative studies of white matter. II. Enzymes involved in triose phosphate metabolism. *Journal of General Physiology* 1964; 47:419.

McEwen, B.S., Stellar, E.: Stress and the individual: Mechanisms leading to disease. *Archives of Internal Medicine* 1993; 153:2093-2101.

McFarland, R.A.: The epidemiology of motor vehicle accidents. *Journal of the American Medical Association* 1962; 180:289-292.

McGregor, S.J., Brown, D., Brock, J.H.: Transferrin-gallium binding in Alzheimer's disease. *The Lancet* 1991; 338:1394-1395.

McMurray, S.: Cleaning up. *The Wall Street Journal* June 11, 1991, pp.A-1, A-6.

McWhorter, W., White, L.: Risk factors for dementia in a national longitudinal study: Preliminary findings. Presented to a NIMH workshop, Bethesda, 1987. Cited by Henderson (1990).

Megalli, M., Freidman, A.: *Masks of Deception: Corporate Front Groups in America.* Essential Information, Washington, D.C., 1991.

Melchior, J.C., Ragaud, D., Colas-Linhart, N., et al; Immunoreactive beta-endorphin increases after an aspartame chocolate drink in healthy human subjects. *Physiology & Behavior* 1991; 50:941-944.

Mendez, M.F., et al: Potential risk factors in Alzheimer's disease: Clinical pathological evidence in 557 brains from the Ramsey Dementia Brain Bank. (Abstract) *Neurology* 1991; 41(Suppl.1):323.

Mesulam, M.-M., Geula, C., Maran, M.A.: Anatomy of cholinesterase inhibition in Alzheimer's disease. *Annals of Neurology* 1987; 22:683-691.

Mesulam, M.-M., Carson, K., Geula, C.: Vessel-bound cholinesterase in the amyloid angiopathy of Alzheimer's disease. (Abstract) *Neurology* 1991; 41(Suppl.1):156.

Metz, R., Surmaczynska, B., Berger, S., Sobel, G.: Glucose tolerance, plasma insulin and free fatty acids in elderly subjects. *Annals of Internal Medicine* 1966; 64:1042.

Metzenbaum, H.: Discussion of S.1557 (Aspartame Safety Act). *Congressional Record-Senate* 1985; August 1, p.S10820.

Metzenbaum, H.M.: Statement for Committee on Labor and Human Resources, *NutraSweet: Health and Safety Concerns* United States Senate, November 3, 1987. 83-178, U.S. Government Printing Office, Washington, 1988, 1-3.

Miller, K.: Attention-deficit disorder affects adults, but some doctors question how widely. *The Wall Street Journal* January 11, 1993, B-1.

Millichap, J.G.: *Environmental Poisons in Our Food.* PNB Publishers, Chicago, 1993.

Mohide, E.A.: Informal care of community-dwelling patients with Alzheimer's disease: Focus on the family caregiver. *Neurology* 1993; 43(Suppl.4):S-16-19.

Montagna, P., et al: Mitochondrial abnormalities in migraine. Preliminary findings. *Headache* 1988; 28:477-480.

Montagna, P., Cortelli, P., Monari, L., et al: ^{31}P-magnetic resonance spectroscopy in migraine without aura. *Neurology* 1994; 44:666-669.

Mooradian, A.D., Garbau, G., Uko-Eninn, A.: In situ quantitation of the age-related and diabetes-related changes in cerebral endothelial barrier antigen. *Clinical Research* 1993; 41:9A.

Morris, J.C., Cole, M., Banker, B.Q., Wright, D.: Hereditary dysphasic dementia and the Pick-Alzheimer spectrum. *Annals of Neurology* 1984; 16:455-466.

Morris, J.C., et al: Very mild Alzheimer's disease: Informant-based clinical, psychometric, and pathologic distention from normal aging. *Neurology* 1991; 41:469-478.

Mortimer, J.A.: Epidemiology of dementia: Cross-cultural comparisons. In *Advances in Neurology. Volume 51: Alzheimer's Disease,* edited by R. J. Wurtman et al. Raven Press, Ltd., New York, 1990, pp.27-33.

Mortimer, J.A., Ebbitt, B., Jun, S., Finch, M.D.: Predictors of cognitive and functional progression in patients with probable Alzheimer's disease. *Neurology* 1992; 42:1689-1696.

Mortimer, J.A., Graves, A.B.; Education and other socioeconomic determinants of dementia and Alzheimer's disease. *Neurology* 1993; 43(Suppl.4):S-39-44.

Moyers, B.: *Healing and the Mind.* Doubleday, New York, 1993.

Murphy, M.: The molecular pathogenesis of Alzheimer's disease: Clinical prospects. *The Lancet* 1992; 340:1512-1515.

Murrell, J., Farlow, M., Ghetti, D., Benson, M.D.: A mutation in the amyloid precursor protein associated with hereditary Alzheimer's disease. *Science* 1991; 254:97-99.

Natelson, B.H., Brassloff, I., Lee, H., Cohen, J.: MR imaging in patients with the chronic fatigue syndrome (CFS). (Abstract) *Neurology* 1993; 43:A272.

National Research Council, Board of Environmental Studies and Toxicology: *Workshop on Health Risk from Exposure to Common Indoor Household Products in Allergic or Chemically Diseased Persons.* 1987; July 1.

National Research Council: *Environmental Neurotoxicology.* National Academy Press, Washington, D.C., 1991, 4.

Nee, L.E., Eldridge, R., Sunderland, T., et al: Dementia of the Alzheimer type: Clinical and family study of 22 twin pairs. *Neurology* 1986; 36:359-363.

Needleman, H.L.: *Human Lead Exposure.* CRC Press, Inc., Boca Raton (Florida), 1992.

Neel, J.V., Fajans, S.S., Conn, J.W., Davidson, R.T.: Diabetes mellitus. In *Genetics and the Epidemiology of Chronic Diseases,* cited by J. V. Neel, M. W. Shaw and W. J. Schull. Public Health Service Publication No. 1163, Washington, D.C., 1965; February.

Nelson, G. Food Protection Act of 1972. *Congressional Record-Senate.* 1972; February 14: No. 18.

Neri, L.C., Hewitt, D.: Aluminium, Alzheimer's disease, and drinking water. *The Lancet* 1991; 338:390.

New York Academy of Sciences: *Neurotoxins and Neurodegenerative Disease.* Edited by J. W. Langston and A. B. Young. Annals of the New York Academy of Sciences 1992; Volume 648.

Noah, T.: EPA study finds unsafe lead levels in 819 water systems across the U.S. *The Wall Street Journal* 1993; May 12: A-2.

Null, G.: Mercury dental amalgams—analyzing the debate. *Townsend Letter for Doctors* 1992; August/September: 762-770.

O'Connor, D.W., et al: Do general practitioners miss dementia in elderly patients? *British Medical Journal* 1988; 299:1107-1110.

Oken, B.S., Kishiyama, S.S., Kaye, J.A.: Attention deficit in Alzheimer's disease is not simulated by antihistamine/anticholinergic drug. (Abstract) *Neurology* 1993; 43:A345.

Olney, J.W., Ho, O.L., Rhee, V.: Brain-damaging potential of protein hydrolysates. *New England Journal of Medicine* 1973; 289:391-393.

Olney, J.W., Labruyere, J., Price, M.T.: Pathological changes induced in cerebral cerebrocortical neurons by phencyclidine and related drugs. *Science* 1989; 244:1360-1362.

Olney, J.W.: Analysis of Adverse Reactions to Monosodium Glutamate. Testimony to Federation of American Societies for Experimental Biology, Bethesda, 1993; April 8.

O'Neill, D.: Physicians, elderly drivers, and dementia. *The Lancet* 1992; 339:41-43.

Ortiz, F.J., Herman, W.A., Smith, M.J., Halter, J.B.: Diminished hypoglycemia counterregulation in older adults. *Clinical Research* 1992; 40: 195A.

Ott, J.N.: *Health and Light.* The Devin-Adair Company, Old Greenwich, Connecticut, 1973.

Ownby, J.H., et al: Scopolamine-induced cerebral metabolic dysfunction does not resemble Alzheimer's disease. (Abstract) *Neurology* 1991; 41(Suppl.1):405.

Panchalingam, K., et al: In vivo ^{31}P NMR shows decreased brain ATP utilization is correlated with severity of dementia in Alzheimer's disease. (Abstract) *Neurology* 1991; 41(Suppl.1):269.

a. Pardridge, W.M.: The safety of aspartame. *Journal of the American Medical Association* 1987; 258:206.

b. Pardridge, W.M.: Phenylalanine transport at the human blood-brain barrier. In *Proceedings of the First International Meeting on Dietary Phenylalanine and Brain Function,* edited by R. J. Wurtman and E. Ritter-Walker, Washington, D.C., 1987; May 8-10: 57-69.

Parker, R.S.: It's enough to make you mad. *Tropic Magazine.* 1973; August 5: 8.

Pasquier, F., Ball, L., Lebert, F., et al: Determination of medial temporal lobe atrophy in early Alzheimer's disease with computed tomography. *The Lancet* 1994; 343:861-862.

Passwater, R.A.: *The Longevity Factor.* Keats Publishing Inc., New Canaan, 1993.

Payan, I.L., et al: Altered aspartate in Alzheimer's neurofibrillary tangles. *Neurochemical Research* 1992; 17:187-191.

Peacock, M.L., Warren, J.T., Jr., Murman, D.L., et al: Novel mutation in codon 665(Glu→Asp) in the amyloid precursor protein (APP) in a patient with late-onset Alzheimer's disease (AD). (Abstract) *Neurology* 1993; 43:A317.

Perl, D.P., Brody, A.R.: Alzheimer's disease: X-ray spectrometric evidence of aluminum accumulation in neurofibrillary tangle-bearing neurons. *Science* 1980; 207:297-299.

Perl, D.P., et al: Intraneuronal aluminum accumulation in amyotrophic lateral sclerosis and parkinsonism-dementia of Gaum. *Science* 1982; 217:1053-1055.

Perls, T., Lipsitz, L., Ooi, W., et al: Preservation of cognitive function in very old men: Effect of selective survival. *Clinical Research* 1992; 40:226A.

Perry, R.H., et al: Cortical cholingeric deficit in mentally impaired parkinsonian patients. *The Lancet* 1983; 309:789-790.

Petersen, R.C., Smith, G.E., Ivnik, R.J., et al: Memory function in very early Alzheimer's disease. *Neurology* 1994; 44:867-872.

Plotnikoff, N.P., Murgo, A., Faith, R.E., Wybran, J.: *Stress and Immunity.* CRC Press, Inc., Boca Raton (Florida), 1992.

Poirier, J., Davignon, J., Bouthillier, D., et al: Apolipoprotein E polymorphism and Alzheimer's disease. *The Lancet* 1993; 342:697-699.

Poldinger, W., Sutter, W.: The influence of psychotropic drugs on driving skill. (German) *Pharmakopsychiatrie Neuro-Psychopharmakologic* 1968; 1:223.

Pozza, G., Chidini, A.: Insulin antagonism in human serum. *The Lancet* 1968; 2:831.

Procter, A.W., Palmer, A.M., Stratmann, G.C., Bowen, D.M.: Glutamate/aspartame-releasing neurones in Alzheimer's disease. *New England Journal of Medicine* 1986; 314:1711-1712.

Quastel, J.H., Tennenbaum, M., Wheatley, A.H.M.: Choline ester formation in, and choline esterase activities of, tissues in vitro. *Biochemistry Journal* 1936; 30:1668.

Rabizadeh, S., Oh, J., Zhong, L., et al: Induction of apoptosis by the low-affirmity NGF receptor. *Science* 1993; 261:345-348.

Randolph, T., Moss, R.: *An Alternative Approach to Allergies* Lippicott & Crowell, New York, 1980.

Randolph, T.: *Environmental Medicine: Beginnings and Bibliographies of Clinical Ecology* Clinical Ecology Publications, Fort Collins, Colorado, 1987.

Ravishankara, A.R., Solomon, S., Turnipseed, A.A., Warren R.F.: Atmospheric lifetimes of long-lived halogenated species. *Sciences* 1993; 259:194-199.

Reaven, G.M., Thompson, L.W., Nahum, D., Haskins, E.: Relationshipp between hyperglycemia and cognitive function in older NIDDM patients. *Diabetes Care* 1990; 13:16-21.

Regland, B., Gottfries, C.: The role of amyloid β-protein in Alzheimer's disease. *The Lancet* 1992; 340:467-469.

Reichlin, S.: Neuroendocrine-immune interactions. *New England Journal of Medicine* 1993; 329:1246-1253.

Reif-Lehrer, L.: Possible significance of adverse reactions to glutamate in humans. *Federation Proceedings* 1976; 35;2205-2211.

Reitano, G., Distefano, G., Vigo, R., et al: Effect of priming of amino acids on insulin and growth hormone response in the premature infant. *Diabetes* 1978; 27:334-337.

Ribak, C.E., Joubran, C., Kesslak, J.P., Bakay, R.A.: A selective decrease in the number of GABAergic somata occurs in pre-seizing monkeys with alumina gel granuloma. *Epilepsy Research* 1989; 4:126-138.

Ribicoff, A.S.: *Chemicals and the Future of Man.* The U.S. Senate Subcommittee on Executive Reorganization and Government Research, Committee on Government Operations, 1971; April 6:1-2.

Riggs, J.E.: Smoking and Alzheimer's disease: protective effect or differential survival bias? *The Lancet* 1993; 342:793-794.

Rizzo, T., Metzger, B.E., Burns, W.J., Burns, K.: Correlations between antepartum maternal metabolism and intelligence of offspring. *New England Journal of Medicine* 1991; 325:911-916.

Rizzo, W.B.; Lorenzo's oil—hope and disappointment. *New England Journal of Medicine* 1993; 329:801-802.

Roberts, G.W., Gentleman, S.M., Lynch, A., Graham, D.I.: βA4 amyloid protein deposition in brain after head trauma. *The Lancet* 1991; 338:1422-1423.

Roberts, H.J.: *Difficult Diagnosis: A Guide to the Interpretation of Obscure Illness.* W. B. Saunders Co., Philadelphia, 1958.

a. Roberts, H.J.: The syndrome of narcolepsy and diabetogenic hyperinsulinism in the American Negro: Its relationship to diabetes mellitus, obesity, dysrhythmias and accelerated cardiovascular disease. *Journal of the National Medical Association* 1964; 56:18-42.

b. Roberts, H.J.: The syndrome of narcolepsy and diabetogenic ("functional") hyperinsulinism, with special reference of obesity, diabetes, idiopathic edema, cerebral dysrhythmias and multiple sclerosis (200 patients). *Journal of the American Geriatrics Society* 1964; 12;926-976.

c. Roberts, H.J.: Chronic refractory fatigue - an "organic" perspective: With emphasis upon the syndrome of narcolepsy and diabetogenic hyperinsulinism. *Medical Times* 1964; 92:1144-1160.

d. Roberts, H.J.: Afternoon glucose tolerance testing: A key to the pathogenesis, early diagnosis and prognosis of diabetogenic hyperinsulinism. *Journal of the American Geriatrics Society* 1964; 12:423-472.

e. Roberts, H.J.: Fatigue as an elusive organic problem. *Consultant* 1964; 4(May):30-34.

a. Roberts, H.J.: Spontaneous leg cramps and "restless legs" due to diabetogenic hyperinsulinism: Observations on 131 patients. *Journal of the American Geriatrics Society* 1965; 13:602-638.

224

c. Roberts, H.J.: Café-au-lait spots (CALS), localized hypomelanosis (LH), and the white forelock (WF) - clues to the syndrome of narcolepsy and diabetogenic hyperinsulinism. *Clinical Research* 1965; 13:267.

a. Roberts, H.J.: The role of diabetogenic hyperinsulinism in the pathogenesis of prostatic hyperplasia and malignancy. *Journal of the American Geriatrics Society* 1966; 14:795-825.

b. Roberts, H.J.: An inquiry into the pathogenesis, rational treatment and prevention of multiple sclerosis, with emphasis upon the combined role of diabetogenic hyperinsulinism and recurrent edema. *Journal of the American Geriatrics Society* 1966; 14:586-608.

c. Roberts, H.J.: On the etiology, rational treatment and prevention of multiple sclerosis. *Southern Medical Journal* 1966; 59:940-950.

d. Roberts, H.J.: Medical disorders and traffic accidents. *New England Journal of Medicine* 1966; 274:915.

e. Roberts, H.J.: Chronic fatigue: psychologic or organic? *Issues of Current Medical Practice* 1966; 3(April):31-35.

f. Roberts, H.J.: Narcolepsy following injury by electric current (3 cases), with commentary on the contributory role of diabetogenic hyperinsulinism. *Archives of Environmental Health* 1966; 13:125-130.

a. Roberts, H.J.: The role of diabetogenic hyperinsulinism in nocturnal angina pectoris, with special reference to the etiology of ischemic heart disease. *Journal of the American Geriatrics Society* 1967; 15:545-555.

b. Roberts, H.J.: Obesity due to the syndrome of narcolepsy and diabetogenic hyperinsulinism: Clinical and therapeutic observations on 252 patients. *Journal of the American Geriatrics Society* 1967; 15:721-743.

c. Roberts, H.J.: The pathogenesis of prostatic hyperplasia and neoplasia. *Geriatrics* 1967; 22:85-92.

d. Roberts, H.J.: Migraine and related vascular headaches due to diabetogenic hyperinsulinism: Observations on pathogenesis and rational treatment in 421 patients. *Headache* 1967; 7:41-62.

Roberts, H.J.: The value of afternoon glucose tolerance testing in the diagnosis, prognosis and rational treatment of "early chemical diabetes": a 5-year experience. *Acta Diabetologica Latina* 1968; 5:532-565.

a. Roberts, H.J.: Hyperthyroidism and thyroiditis precipitated by severe caloric restriction: Report of 8 cases. Abstract 305. Program of the 51st meeting, Endocrine Society, New York, 1969; June 27.

b. Roberts, H.J.: A clinical and metabolic re-evaluation of reading disability. In *Selected Papers on Learning Disabilities. 5th Annual Conference, Association for Children with Learning Disabilities.* Academic Therapy Publications, San Raphael, California, 1969, 472-490.

Roberts, H.J.: Overlooked dangers of weight reduction. *Medical Counterpoint* 1970; 2 September: 14-21.

a. Roberts, H.J.: The role of pathologic drowsiness in traffic accidents: An epidemiologic study. *Tufts Medical Alumni Bulletin* 1971; 32:32-41.

b. Roberts, H.J.: *The Causes, Ecology and Prevention of Traffic Accidents.* Charles C Thomas, Springfield, 1971.

Roberts, H.J.: Spontaneous leg cramps and "restless legs" due to diabetogenic (functional) hyperinsulinism. *Journal of the Florida Medical Association* 1973; 60:29-31.

a. Roberts, H.J.: *Is Vasectomy Safe? Medical, Public Health and Legal Implications.* Sunshine Academic Press, West Palm Beach, 1979.

b. Roberts, H.J.: Thrombophlebitis associated with vitamin E therapy: With a commentary on other medical side effects. *Angiology* 1979; 30:169-176.

a. Roberts, H.J.: Dolomite as a source of toxic metals. *New England Journal of Medicine* 1981; 30:423.

b. Roberts, H.J.: More on dolomite. *New England Journal of Medicine* 1981; 304:1367.

c. Roberts, H.J.: Perspective on vitamin E as therapy. *Journal of the American Medical Association* 1981; 246:129-131.

a. Roberts, H.J.: Timed repetitive ankle jerk responses in early diabetic neuropathy. *Southern Medical Journal* 1982; 75:411-416.

a. Roberts, H.J.: Potential toxicity due to dolomite and bonemeal. *Southern Medical Journal* 1983; 76:556-559.

b. Roberts, H.J.: The vitamin E enigma: Perspectives for physicians. Chapter 26 in *Controversies in Dermatology,* edited by E. Epstein, W. B. Saunders Co., Philadelphia, 1984; 366-394.

Roberts, H.J.: The hazards of very-low-calorie dieting. *American Journal of Clinical Nutrition* 1985; 41:171-172.

Roberts, H.J.: Respiratory hazards of anti-static clothes softeners. *Palm Beach County Medical Society Bulletin* 1986; January:24-31.

Roberts, H.J.: Neurologic, psychiatric and behavioral reactions to aspartame in 505 aspartame reactions. In *Proceedings of the First International Conference on Dietary Phenylalanine and Brain Function,* edited by R.J. Wurtman and E. Ritter-Walker, Washington, D.C., 1987; May 8-10:477-481.

d. Roberts, H.J.: The Aspartame Problem. Statement for Committee on Labor and Human Resources, U.S. Senate, *Hearing on "NutraSweet"—Health and Safety Concerns.* Novermber 3, 1987. 83-178, U.S. Government Printing Office, Washington, 1988:466-467.

e. Roberts, H.J.: Reactions attributed to aspartame-containing products: 551 cases. *Journal of Applied Nutrition* 1988; 40:85-94.

Roberts, H.J.: *Aspartame (NutraSweet*): Is It Safe? Philadelphia,* The Charles Press, 1989.

Roberts, H.J.: Pentachlorophenol-associated aplastic anemia, red cell aplasia, leukemia and other blood disorders. *Journal of the Florida Medical Association* 1990; 77:86-90.

a. Roberts, H.J.: Aspartame-associated confusion and memory loss. *Townsend Letter for Doctors* 1991; June:442-443.

b. Roberts, H.J.: Syndrome(s) X. *The Lancet* 1991; 337:916-917.

a. Roberts, H.J.: Aspartame: Is it safe? Interview with H. J. Roberts, M.D. *Mastering Food Allergies* 1992; 7 (#1):3-6.

b. Roberts, H.J.: *Sweet'ner Dearest: Bittersweet Vignettes About Aspartame (NutraSweet©).* Sunshine Sentinel Press, West Palm Beach, 1992.

c. Roberts, H.J.: Re: Toxicology of fluoride. *Townsend letter for Doctors* 1992; July, 623-624.

d. Roberts, H.J.: Chronic fatigue. *Townsend Letter for Doctors* 1992; August/September:742.

Roberts, H.J.: Analysis of Adverse Reactions to Monosodium Glutamate. Testimony to Federation of American Societies for Experimental Biology, Bethesda. 1993; April 8.

Roberts, H.J.: *Mega Vitamin E: Is It Safe?* Sunshine Sentinel Press, West Palm Beach, 1994.

Robertson, J.A., Salusky, I.B., Goodman, W.G., Norris, K.C., Coburn, J.W.: Sucralfate, intestinal aluminum absorption, and aluminum toxicity in a patient on dialysis. *Annals of Internal Medicine* 1989; 111:179-180.

Rocca, W.A., et al: Frequency and distribution of Alzheimer's disease (AD) in Europe: A collaborative study of 1980-1990 prevalence findings. (Abstract) *Neurology* 1991; 41(Suppl.1):372.

Rogers, P.J., Keedwell, P., Blundell, J.E.: Further analysis of the short-term inhibition of food intake in humans by the dipeptide L-aspartyl-L-phenylalanine methyl ester (aspartame). *Physiology & Behavior* 1991; 14:739-743.

Rosenberg, I.H.: Starch blockers—still no calorie-free lunch. *New England Journal of Medicine* 1982; 307:1444-1445.

Rosenberg, I.H., Miller, J.W.: Nutritional factors in physical and cognitive functions of elderly people. *American Journal of Clinical Nutrition* 1992; 55(Suppl.6):1237-1243.

Rosenberg, N.L., et al: 1.5 Tesla MRI bindings in toluene patients. (Abstract) *Neurology* 1991; 41(Suppl.1):237.

Rosenstock, L., Keifer, M., Daniell, W.E., et al: Chronic central nervous system effects of acute organophosphate pesticide intoxication. *The Lancet* 1991; 338:223-236.

Rosenthal, E.: New cautions on dental anesthesia. *The New York Times* 1993; June 16:B-7.

Roses, A.D., Strittmatter, W.J., Pericak-Vance, M.A., et al: Clinical application of apolipoprotein E genotyping to Alzheimer's disease. *The Lancet* 1994; 343:1564-1565.

Rowland, A.S., Baird, D.D., Weinberg, C.R., et al: Reduced fertility among women employed as dental assistants exposed to high levels of nitrous oxide. *New England Journal of Medicine* 1992; 327:933-997.

Roznoski, M.M., Huang, S., Burns, R.: Phenylalanine interferes with metabolism of exogenous L-dopa at the cell level. (Abstract) *Neurology* 1993; 43:A195.

Rummaus, T.A., Davis, L.J., Jr., Morse, R.M., Ivnik, R.J.: Learning and memory impairment in older, detoxified, benzodiazepine-dependent patients. *Mayo Clinic Proceedings* 1993; 68:731-737.

Salganik, I., Korczyn, A.: Risk factors for dementia in Parkinson's disease. *Advances in Neurology* 1990; 53:343-347.

Salusky, I.B., et al: Aluminum accumulation in patients with chronic renal disease. (Letter) *New England Journal of Medicine* 1991; 325:208-209.

Samuels, A.: *MSG: A Review of the Literature and Critique of Industry Sponsored Research.* Private printing. 1991; July 1.

Samuels, J.L.: Evaluation of the safety of amino acids and related products. Presentation to Life Sciences Research Office, Federation of American Societies for Experimental Biology, Docket No. 90N-0379, 1991; February 4.

Sanz, P., Amorors, E., Prat, A., et al: Aluminium exposure in children associated with industrial waste. (Letter) *The Lancet* 1992; 339:1488-1489.

Sapira, J.D.: Dysphoria and impaired mentation in young physicians. *Southern Medical Journal* 1977; 70:1305-1307.

Sapolsky, R.M.: *Stress, the Aging Brain, and the Mechanisms of Neuron Death.* MIT Press, Cambridge, 1992.

Sarafian, T.A., Verity, M.A.: Changes in protein phosphorylation in cultured neurons after exposure to methyl mercury. *Annals of the New York Academy of Sciences* 1993; 679:65-77.

Schapira, R., Chou, C.-H.: Differential racemization of aspartate and serine in human myelin basic protein. *Biochemical and Biophysiology Research Communications* 1987; 146:1342-1349.

a. Scheltens, P., et al: Hippocampal atrophy on magnetic resonance imaging in Alzheimer's Disease and normal aging. (Abstract) *Neurology* 1991; 41(Suppl.1):341.

b. Scheltens, P., et al: Sleep apnea syndrome presenting with cognitive impairment. *Neurology* 1991; 41:155-156.

Schlenker, T.L., Fritz, C.J., Mark, D., et al: Screening for pediatric lead poisoning. *Journal of the American Medical Association* 1994; 271-1346-1348.

Schlettwein-Gsell, D.: Nutrition and the quality of life: a measure for the outcome of nutritional intervention? *American Journal of Clinical Nutrition* 1992; 55(Suppl.6): 1263-1266.

Schoenberg, B.S., Anderson, D.A., Haerer, A.F.: Severe dementia: Prevalence and clinical features in a biracial U.S. population. *Archives of Neurology* 1985; 42:740-743.

Segal, S.: Disorders of Galactose Metabolism. Chapter 13 in *The Metabolic Basis of Inherited Disease,* 6th Edition, edited by C. R. Scriver, A. L. Beaudet, W. S. Sly, and D. Valle, Mc-Graw Hill Information Services Co., New York, 1989:453-480.

Selhub, J., Jacques, P.F., Wilson, P.W.F., Rush, D., Rosenberg, I.H.: Vitamin status and intake as primary determinants of homocysteinemia in an elderly population. *Journal of the American Medical Association* 1993; 270:2693-2698.

Seltzer, B., Sherwin, I.: A comparison of clinical features of early and late onset primary degenerative dementia: One entity or two? *Archives of Neurology* 1983; 40:143-146.

Semchuk, K.M., Love, E.J., Lee, R.G.: Parkinson's disease and exposure to agricultural work and pesticide chemicals. *Neurology* 1992; 42:1328-1335.

Sengstock, G., Alanow, C.W., Arendash, G.: Iron infusion into the substantia nigra induces progressive reduction in striatal dopamine. (Abstract) *Neurology* 1993; 43:A389.

Shaffer, M.: Cell death opens vistas in cancer and Alzheimer's research. *Medical World News* 1993; May: 32, 41.

Shalat S.L.: Risk factors for Alzheimer's disease: Fact of theory? *Geriatric Medicine Today* 1989; 8 (March): 26-47.

Shannon, M., Graef, J.: Hazard of lead in infant formula. *New England Journal of Medicine* 1992; 326:137.

Shima, K., Foa, P.F.: Serum immunoreacting insulin and free fatty acid responses to oral glucose and to intravenous tolbutamide in normal, prediabetic and diabetic subjects. *Excerpta Medica Proceedings Book Lodge Symposium* (International Congress Series) 1967; 149:217.

Sibbison, J.B.: USA: Science and senility. *The Lancet* 1991; 338:176-177.

Siddique, T., et al: Linkage of a gene causing familial amyotrophic lateral sclerosis to chromosome 21 and evidence of genetic-locus heterogeneity. *New England Journal of Medicine* 1991; 324:1381-1384.

Simonian, N.A., Hyman, B.T.: Cytochrome oxidase is altered in the hippocampal formation in Alzheimer's disease. (Abstract) *Neurology* 1993; 43:A251.

Singh, M., Simpkins, J.W.: The effect of estradiol deprivation and replacement on high affinity choline uptake in frontal cortex and hippocampus of female Sprague Dawley rats. (Abstract 1263) 75th Annual Meeting of the Endocrine Society, Las Vegas, 1993; June 9.

Skoog, I., Nilsson, L., Palmertz, B., et al: A population-based study of dementia in 85-year-olds. *New England Journal of Medicine* 1993; 328:153-158.

Skow, J.: Can lawns be justified? *Time* 1991; June 3:63-64.

Smith, B.L.: Organic foods vs supermarket foods: Element levels. *Journal of Applied Nutrition* 1993; 45(#1): 35-39.

Snowdon, D.A., Astwald, S.K., Keenan, N.K., et al: Years of life with good and poor mental and physical function in the elderly. *Journal of Clinical Epidemiology* 1989; 42:1055-1066.

Spears, G.: U.S. wants lead tests for all kids. *The Miami Herald* October 2, 1991, pp. A-1, A-16.

Spencer, P.S., et al: Guam amyotrophic lateral sclerosis parkinsonism-dementia linked to a plant excitant neurotoxin. *Science* 1987; 237:517-522.

Spiers, P., Schomer, D., Sabounjian, L.: Aspartame and human behavior: cognitive and behavioral observations. In *Proceedings of the First International Meeting on Dietary Phenylalanine and Brain Function,* edited by R. J. Wurtman and E. Ritter-Walker, Washington, D.C., 1987; May 8-10:193-206.

Stacher, G.: Satiety effect of cholecystokinin and ceruletide in lean and obese men. In *Neuronal Cholecystokinin,* edited by J. Vanderhaeghen and J. N. Crawley, *Annals of the New York Academy of Sciences* 1985; 448:431-436.

Steiner, D.F., Ohagi, S., Nagamatsu, S., Bell, G.I., Nishi, M.: Is islet amyloid polypeptide a significant factor in pathogenesis or pathophysiology of diabetes? *Diabetes* 1991; 40:305-309.

Stern, Y., Marder, K., Sano, M., et al: Educational and occupational attainment: Risk factors for incident dementia. (Abstract) *Neurology* 1993; 43:A234.

Stern, Y., Gurland, B., Tatemichi, T.K., et al: Influence of education and occupation on the incidence of Alzheimer's disease. *Journal of the American Medical Association* 1994; 271:1004-1010.

Stevenson, H.W., Chen, C., Lee, S.: Mathematics achievement of Chinese, Japanese, and the American children: Ten years later. *Science* 1993; 259:53-58.

Stipp, D.: Heart-attack study adds to the cautions about iron in the diet. *The Wall Street Journal* September 8, 1992, A-1, 9.

Stone, A.: Cited by D. Goleman. *The New York Times* May 11, 1994, B-6.

Stone, R.: New marker for nerve damage. *Science* 1993; 259;1541.

Sunderland, T.: Cited by *Medical World News* April 1991, 20.

Swanson, J.E., Laine, D.C., Thomas, W., Bantle, J.P.: Metabolic effects of dietary fructose in healthy subjects. *American Journal of Clinical Nutrition* 1992, 55:851-856.

Szanto, S.: Elevated insulin levels seen in heavy smokers. *Diabetes Outlook* 1968; 3 (October): 4.

Szasz, T.: Diagnoses are not diseases. *The Lancet* 1991; 338;1574-1576.

Tallal, P.: Cited by *The Wall Street Journal* 1992; October 29: B-12.

Tamminga, C.A., Lucignani, G., Porrino, L.J., Chase, T.N.: Cholecystokinin octapeptide's effect on local cerebral glucose utilization in the laboratory rat. In *Neuronal Cholecystokinin,* edited by J. Vanderhaeghen and J. N. Crawley, *Annals of the New York Academy of Sciences* 1985; 448;663-665.

Tapanainen, P.J., Bang, P., Vreman, H.: Effect of maternal hypoxia on insulin-like growth factors and their binding proteins in the rat fetus. (Abstract 887) 75th Annual Meeting of the Endocrine Society, Las Vegas, June 9, 1993.

Tendler, D.A., et al: Effect of MK-801 on excitatory and inhibitory amino acids during hypoxia and seizure: In vivo cerebral microdialysis study. (Abstract) *Neurology* 1991; 41(Suppl.1):414.

Tennakone, K., Wickramanayake, S.: Aluminum leaching from cooking utensils. *Nature* 1987; 325:202.

Terry, R.D., Masliah, E., Salmon, D.T., et al: Physical basis of cognitive alterations in Alzheimer's disease: Synapse loss in the major correlate of cognitive impairment. *Annals of Neurology* 1991; 30:572-580.

Thayer, A.M.: Use of specialty food additives to continue to grow. *Chemical & Engineering News* 1991; June 3: 9-12.

Thomison, J.B.: Mens sana in corpore sano. *Southern Medical Journal* 1983: 76:1-2.

Thompson, A.J., et al: Magnetic resonance imaging changes in early treated patients with phenylketonuria. *The Lancet* 1991; 337:1224.

228

Tocci, P.M., Beber, B.: Anomalous phenylalanine loading responses in relation to cleft lip and cleft palate. *Pediatrics* 1973; 52;109.

Tolchin, M.: Frequent fliers saying fresh air is awfully thin at 30,000 feet. *The New York Times* 1993; June 6:1,15.

Tollefson, L., Barnard, R.J., Glinsmann, W.H.: Monitoring of adverse reactions to aspartame reported to the U.S. Food and Drug Administration. In *Proceedings of the First International Meeting on Dietary Phenylalanine and Brain Function,* edited by R. J. Wurtman and E. Ritter-Walker, Washington, D.C. 1987; May 8-10:347-372.

Tsou, V.M., et al: Elevated plasma aluminum levels in normal infants receiving antacids containing aluminum. *Pediatrics* 1991; 87:148-151.

Turski, L., Meldrum, D.S., Cavalheiro, E.A., et al: Paradoxical anticonvulsant activity of the excitatory amino acid N-methyl-D-aspartate in the rat caudate-putamen. *Proceedings of the National Academy of Sciences* USA 1984; 64:1689-1693.

a. Tuszynski, M.H., Amaral, D.G., Gage, F.H.: Nerve growth factor infusion in the primate brain prevents cholinergic neuron degeneration. (Abstract) **Neurology** 1991; 41(Suppl.1):270.

b. Tuszynski, M.H., Sang, H., Yoshida, K., Gage, F.H.: Recombinant human nerve growth factor infusions prevent cholinergic neuronal degeneration in the adult primate brain. *Annals of Neurology* 1991; 30:625-636.

U.S. Department of Health and Human Services Task Force on Alzheimer's Disease: *Alzheimer's Disease: A Scientific Guide for Health Practitioners.* NIH Publication No. 84-2251, 1984; May.

U.S. Preventive Services Task Force: Routine iron supplementation during pregnancy. Policy statement. *Journal of the American Medical Association* 1993; 270:2946-2854.

Vega, W.A., Kolody, B., Hwang, J., Noble, A.: Prevalence and magnitude of perinatal substance exposures in California. *New England Journal of Medicine* 1993; 329:850-854.

Waldholz, M.: Clue to a killer. *The Wall Street Journal* 1993; June 7: A-1, 6.

Webb, D.: Drinking large quantities of fruit juice can be harmful to babies' development. *The New York Times* 1994; April 6: B-7.

Wecker, L., et al: The aging population. *Journal of the Florida Medical Association* 1991; 78:643-645.

Weiger, W.A.: Chronic fatigue syndrome. (Letter) *Neurology* 1993; 43:1866-1867.

Weir, C.E.: *Benefits from Human Nutrition Research.* Human Nutrition Research Division, United States Department of Agriculture, Washington, D.C., 1971.

Wehmeier, K.R., Mooradiran, A.D.: Antioxidative potential of glucose and other simple carbohydrates. (Abstract 1494) 75th Meeting of the Endocrine Society, Las Vegas, June 9, 1993.

White, D.M., Longstreth, W.T., Rosenstock, L., et al: Neurologic syndrome in 25 workers from an aluminum smelting plant. *Archives of Internal Medicine* 1992; 152:1443-1448.

Willett, W.C., Stampfer, M.J., Manson, J.E., et al: Intake of trans fatty acids and risk of coronary heart disease among women. *The Lancet* 1993; 341:581-585.

Williamson, J.R., Chang, K., Frangos, M., et al: Hyperglycemic pseudohypoxia and diabetic complications. *Diabetes* 1993; 42:801-813.

Wing, R.R., Matthews, K.A., Kuller, L.H., et al: Environmental and familial contributions to insulin levels and change in insulin levels in middle-aged women. *Journal of the American Medical Association* 1992; 268:1890-1895.

Winick, M.: Malnutrition: The time of the insult is critical. *Roche Medical Image & Commentary.* 1969; December:3.

Winick, M.: Nutrition and nerve cell growth. *Federation Proceedings* 1970; 29:1510-1515.

Winslow, R.: Use of birth control pill surges in U.S. *The Wall Street Journal* 1991; August 20:B-4.

Withers, J.J., Woolf, A.S., Kingswood, J.C., Tsang, W.N., Mansell, M.A.: Encephalopathy in patient taking aluminium-containing agents, including sucralfate. *The Lancet* 1989; 334:674.

Wong, R., Lopaschuk, G., Zhu, G., et al: Skeletal muscle metabolism in the chronic fatigue syndrome. *Chest* 1992; 102:1716-1722.

Wurtman, R.J., et al: Choline metabolism in cholinergic neurons: Implications for the pathogenesis of neurodegenerative diseases. In *Advances in Neurology. Volume 51: Alzheimer's Disease,* edited by R. J. Wurtman et al. Raven Press, Ltd., New York, 1990:117-125.

Wurtman, R.: Cited by *The Wall Street Journal* 1993; June 7:A-6.

Xintaras, C., et al: Neurotoxic effects of exposed chemical workers. In *Public Control of Environmental Health Hazards,* edited by E. C. Hammond and I. J. Selikoff. Annals of the New York Academy of Sciences 1979; 329:30-38.

Yakymyshyn, L.Y., Reid, D.W.J., Campbell, D.J.: Problems in the biochemical detection of heterozygotes for phenylketonuria. *Clinical Biochemistry* 1972; 5:73-81.

Yankner, B.A., Kowall, M., Chen, M.: Nerve growth factor is increased in Alzheimer's disease. (Abstract) *Neurology* 1991; 41(Suppl.1):270.

Yazigi, R.A., Odem, R.R., Polakoski, K.L.: Demonstration of specific binding of cocaine to human spermatozoa. *Journal of the American Medical Association* 1991; 266:1956-1959.

Yiamouyiannis, J.: *Fluoride: The Aging Factor.* Health Action Press, Delaware, Ohio, 1986.

Yoshimasu, F., Kokmen, E., Hay, I.D., et al: The association between Alzheimer's disease and thyroid disease in Rochester, Minnesota. *Neurology* 1991; 41:1745-1747.

Young, F., et al: The influence of a family history of asthma and parental smoking on airway responsiveness in early infancy. *New England Journal of Medicine* 1991; 324:1168-1173.

Yudkin, J.: Dietary carbohydrate and ischemic heart disease. *American Heart Journal* 1963; 66;835.

Yudkin, J.: Dietary aspects of atherosclerosis. *Angiology* 1966; 17:127.

Yudkin, J.: Evolutionary and historical changes in dietary carbohydrates. *American Journal of Clinical Nutrition* 1967; 20:108.

Yue- Zhen, H., et al: Syndrome of endemic arsenism and fluorosis: A clinical study. *Chinese Medical Journal* 1992; 105:586-590.

Zaccaria, M., Borea, P.A., Ponchia, A., et al: Effect of high altitude hypoxia on small α2-adrenergic receptors. (Abstract 50) *Annual Meeting of the Endocrine Society,* Las Vegas, 1993; June 6.

Zametkin, A.J., Nordahl, T.E., Gross, M., et al: Cerebral glucose metabolism in adults with hyperactivity of childhood onset. *New England Journal of Medicine* 1990; 323:1361-1366.

Zeytinoglu, I.Y., Gherondache, C.N. Pincus, G.: The process of aging: Serum glucose and immunoreactive insulin levels during the oral glucose tolerance test. *Journal of the American Geriatrics Society* 1969; 17:1-4.

Zweig, R.M., et al: A case of Alzheimer's disease and hippocampal sclerosis with normal cholinergic activity in basal forebrain, neurocortex, and hippocampus. *Neurology* 1989; 39:288-290.

INDEX

232